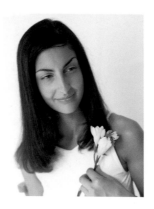

indian
beauty secrets

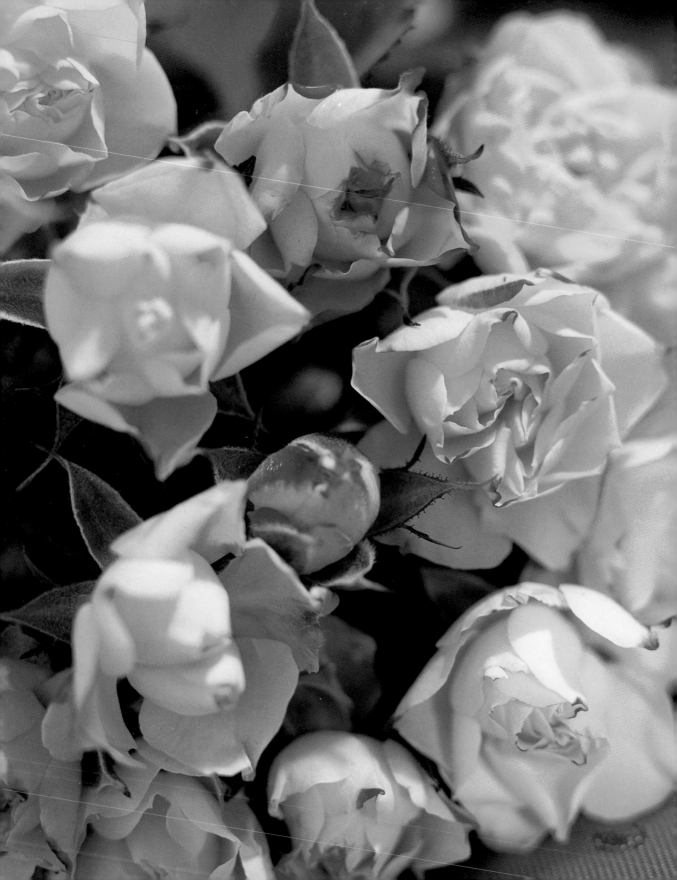

indian
beauty secrets

pamper your body and soul

MONISHA BHARADWAJ

photography by donna eaves

KYLE CATHIE LIMITED

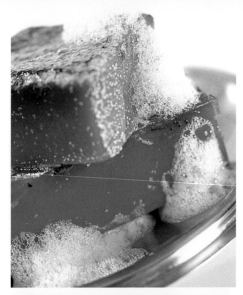

This book is for my husband Nitish who is the perfect man for the woman in me and makes me feel cherished and beautiful every day of our life together, and for my children Arrush and Saayli who are God's most precious and beautiful gifts to us.

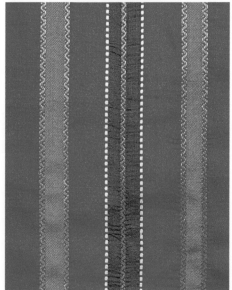

First published in Great Britain in 2000 by

Kyle Cathie Limited

122 Arlington Road, London NW1 7HP

ISBN 1 85626 363 0

Text © 2000 Monisha Bharadwaj

Photography © 2000 Donna Eaves

(See also other copyright acknowledgements on page 160)

Edited by **Sheila Boniface**

Assisted by **Georgina Burns**

Designed by **Mark Latter, Vivid**

Copy edited by **Ruth Baldwin**

Proofread & Indexed by **Tasha Goddard**

Production by **Lorraine Baird and Sha Huxtable**

Monisha Bharadwaj is hereby identified as the author of this work in accordance with Section 77 of the Copyright, Designs and Patents Act 1988

A CIP catalogue record for this title is available from the British Library

Printed and bound in Singapore by Kyodo Printing Co.

Contents

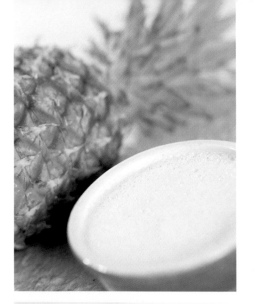

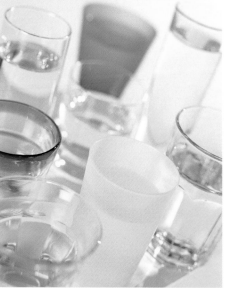

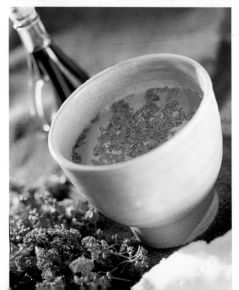

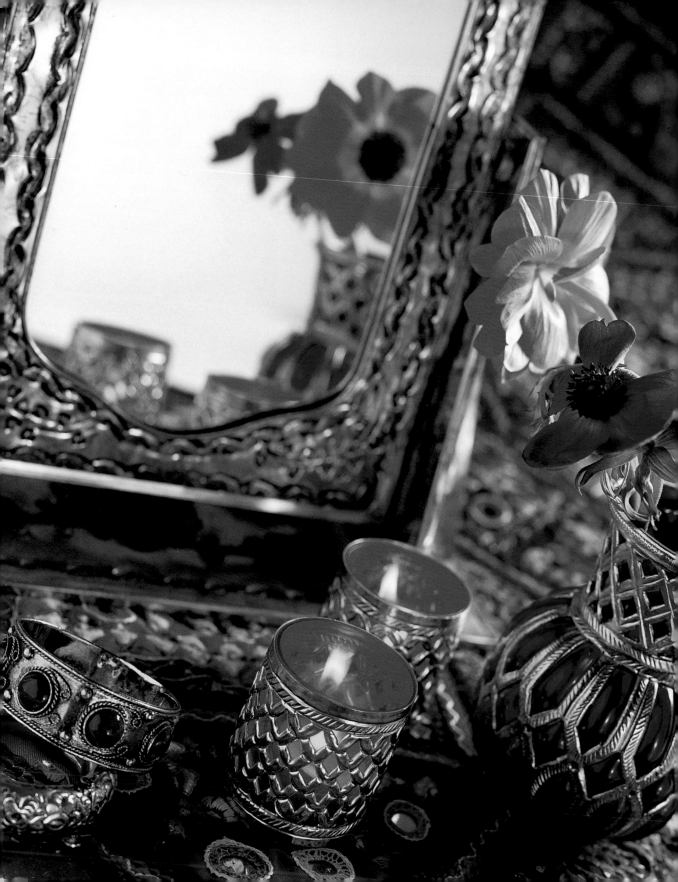

'You are refreshing and vital as the air, graceful and tender as sparkling water, lustrous and consuming as flames of fire, generous and enveloping as space and stable and deep as the earth… you elemental woman are perfect beauty itself.' *ancient essay on 'Panchakanya' or the five elemental women of Indian mythology.*

introduction

Indians have worshipped nature and its power since Vedic times, as far back as 1500 BC. They have understood the awesome energy of water, wind and fire, the limitless vista of earth and space and the gentle, restoring properties of the countless plants that grew in abundance all around them. They used these plants to cure disease and promote health, and to rejuvenate and maintain their skin, hair and eyes. Even in those days beauty was closely associated with the bounty of nature.

The essential knowledge of herbs known as Ayurveda was passed down and refined by many wise and experienced sages. One of the oldest and most revered texts on Ayurveda, the *Charak Samhita*, by the great sage Charak, was written c. AD 150. Even today the life of every Indian is in some way influenced by Ayurveda – from the manner in which they combine foods to the remedies that they remember their grandmothers using for the most gentle but effective relief from everyday health problems.

Ayurveda is also closely linked to beauty. It has been known for thousands of years that the body accepts and responds to natural ingredients more readily than it does to chemicals. Nature itself was the inspiration when thousands of years ago our ancestors searched for perfect beauty. The soft, dewy petals of the rose suggested the prized texture of beautiful skin, the fragrance of the musk-deer as it trotted past became the perfume of a cleansed body, the billowing clouds set an example for long, dark tresses, the sensuous fish became the ideal shape for lovely eyes and the dance of the peacock symbolised grace of movement.

Romantic literature through the centuries is peppered with comparisons of the heroine to various examples in nature, and these lovely women are often shown using natural ingredients on their face and body as if to capture some of the beauty for themselves. Petals in the bath were believed to soften the skin, milk was considered to purify and whiten the body and a stroll in the moonlight was said to give the face a silvery glow.

One of the most beautiful legendary heroines of classical Indian literature, Shakuntala, was born of an *apsara* or celestial water nymph and grew up in the forest with deer

The delicate and luminous Taj Mahal, often described as a poem in marble, was built as a tomb for Queen Mumtaz Mahal and is a symbol of eternal love and beauty. Modern Indian romantic poetry often compares a beautiful woman to its regal loveliness.

and butterflies for friends and tree bark and flowers as her ornaments. When she was a young maiden, Dushyant, the king of the region, spotted her while he was out hunting. He was instantly captivated by her beauty and knew that he had to marry her. His ministers were aghast that he could desire this forest girl when he could have had any princess he wanted. But Dushyant was mesmerised.

The concept of beauty has varied from culture to culture and through the centuries. The ancient Greeks divided the face into three equal parts and considered perfect facial proportions to be the ideal of beauty. The

'Her face, without any cosmetic, still shines like the moon, her full hips and curved waist are all the more enchanting because of her rough bark clothes and her breasts bloom under the swaying garlands of flowers she wears. I care not for the lustre of jewels or the wrapper of silks...'

Kalidasa in Shakuntalam (c. AD 375–454)

Egyptians found beauty in the sculpted features of Queen Nefertiti (c. 1500 BC) and Queen Cleopatra with their high cheekbones and long, graceful necks. Renaissance painters projected beauty as cherubic nymphs with

plump, pink cheeks and flowing, red hair.

However, there is a universal concept of beauty and that, simply put, is clear, radiant skin, sparkling eyes, healthy hair and a positive, self-confident attitude to life. These are the qualities that we all strive for, and these will continue to be sought after by men and women for many centuries to come.

We all add our own extra dimension to this essential concept of beauty. Make-up, hair-dress, the right clothes and personal grooming put a finishing gloss. Archaeologists in the twentieth century believed that the Chinese were the first to discover make-up. Travellers returning to Egypt from China about five thousand years ago took the knowledge back with them, where there is extensive evidence in the form of buried cosmetic jars and make-up tools. Museums with Egyptian collections have displays of kohl pots and sticks for its application, burnished metal plaques used as mirrors, combs crafted out of wood or ivory in the shape of wild animals and birds, and pestles and tiny bowls for mixing cosmetics, some of which still bear traces of these unique mixtures.

The desire to decorate the body and face is as primitive as the early civilisations and can be seen in every land from Africa to Australia. In India, where ornamentation has always been a part of everyday life, it goes without saying that the human form, and more especially the female one, has been an important candidate for decoration. Women all over the world are passionate about beauty, but in India every woman, whether she lives in the dry, dusty desert of Rajasthan or the lush, tropical forests of Kerala, will take special pride in embellishing herself as she does her home and her surroundings. Indian culture from as far back as five thousand years ago has encouraged women to understand and express their sensual self as a natural function. Ancient temples are full of exotic women with large breasts and full thighs engaged in any number of sexual positions. Sensual allure, for the opposite sex as well as for the natural expression of oneself, along with an aura of mystery, has always been the essence of Indian beauty. The *Kamasutra*, India's famous treatise on the subject of sex, written by the sage Vyatsyayan between the first and sixth century AD, also elaborates on how to seduce and keep the interest of the opposite sex by emphasising one's beauty.

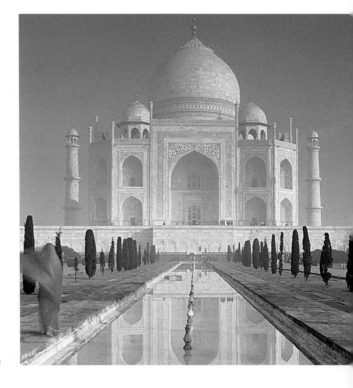

Traditionally, Indian women are not afraid of colour or design. The natural world of India is awash with dazzling, sometimes shocking, hues from hot pink to lime green, so wearing such daring colours does not seem surprising. Also, each region in India has its own particular form of personal decoration, in the way the *bindi* or forehead mark is worn, or in what type of jewellery is fashioned out of gold, silver or gems. In Gujarat, village women will permanently mark their arm with a tattoo of their husband's name and have little blue dots, meant to be beauty marks, tattooed on to their foreheads and chins, whereas a woman from Tamilnadu will adorn herself with three nose rings, one on the left, one on the right and one in the centre through the soft skin under the tip of her nose. In

fact, wise, old women of the south say that these nose rings serve to attract the eye of the beholder to a dazzling smile and the allure of feminine lips!

from mother to daughter

The one thing that is common to the whole of India is that the beauty culture, which is essentially a female world, is based on age-old secrets and the ancient wisdom of past experience. These secrets are a legacy passed down the generations from mother to daughter and beauty routines are set up and practised right from a girl's first few days of

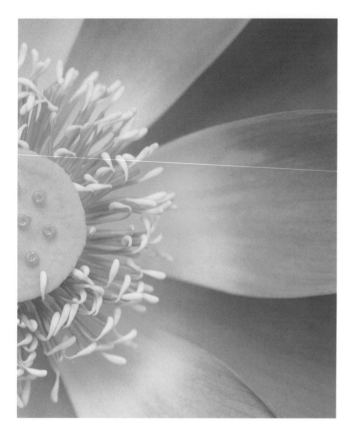

lotions from conversations between her mother, grandmothers, aunts and cousins. She will be taught how to use fruits, herbs, nuts and pulses to polish her skin, fragrance her hair and mouth and soften her feet. She will understand the essentials of Ayurveda – which foods when eaten together create heat in the body and which foods are particularly cooling – and she will grow up with all the knowledge she will need to make the most of her looks. Even today the modern Indian woman still largely follows the familiar beauty routines and advice handed down to her. She still uses natural kitchen ingredients to make her own beauty products, although she will now supplement these with commercial creams and lotions when she is pressed for time.

The beauty secrets of India are for women everywhere. They respond to a universal concept of pure, natural beauty and are easy to follow. They are also based on centuries of experience, are completely natural and they work successfully without any undesirable side-effects. They are as effective for western women as they are within India – from the fair, rosy-cheeked women of the Himalayas to the dark, velvety-skinned beauties of the south.

This book is for women all over the world. It not only reveals the beauty secrets of a vast number of Indian women and their female ancestors, but also relies on the expertise of Ayurveda and ancient Indian herbal beauty

above
The lovely colour, fragrance and shape of a lotus as well as its unique ability to flourish even in the most slimy and dirty water sets an example for all women.

right
Lakshmi, the beautiful goddess of wealth, showers endless coins on her devotees as she stands in a lotus of purity and wisdom.

life. Special care is taken over the skin and hair care of newly born girls – a gentle daily massage with secret mixtures ensures that body hair will gradually fade away in a few months, the head is massaged with rejuvenating oils that promote healthy hair throughout life and the eyes are lined with pure, home-made kohl that thickens the lashes and strengthens vision. This baby girl will grow up listening to stories of valiant heroes and beautiful, courageous women and will learn the secret family recipes for creams, masks and lore to restore, maintain and improve on what nature has given us. It discusses the Indian concepts of meditation, inner peace and positive thinking so that we can all aspire to be calmer, more captivating and certainly more time- and power-efficient.

the indian bride

The beauty rituals learned by a young woman are perhaps of most significance on the day of her wedding when she has to look her radiant best. Nina Epton writes in her book about the queen who inspired the Taj Mahal, *Beloved Empress Mumtaz Mahal*:

'A little before midnight Arjumand (later called Mumtaz Mahal) was given a ritual bath by her mother and various aunts. They escorted her to her bathroom wrapped in white cotton. Her long black hair was loosened, washed and her face bathed with the same herb infused water.

One of her aunts picked up an earthenware jar containing seven little balls of a creamy substance coloured blue, pink, red, green, yellow, white and orange (seven for luck). These were kneaded into a homogenous mask and spread on Arjumand's face, neck and breasts, then washed off with perfumed soap.

…The following morning was taken up with the bridal makeup, which took the palace experts nearly three hours to apply… Gold leaf was applied to her hairline; a golden dragon-fly was impressed upon her forehead on a wax background. Her eyes were heavily underlined with kohl and prolonged by upward slanting strokes of the brush.'

Each region of India has its own typical bridal make-up and attire. Although every bride has a ritual bath with herbs and milk, geography and local customs determine how she will be dressed. In Punjab, she wears red, her wrists are covered in ivory bangles stained red and the parting of her hair is decorated with a gold ornament called the *tikka*. Her palms and feet are embellished with beautiful henna patterns. In the south she wears yellow silk, ruby- and emerald-encrusted jewellery and a wide, gold belt with figures of Lakshmi, the goddess of wealth and prosperity, on her waist. Her hair is woven with countless garlands of tiny, fragrant flowers. In Maharashtra the bride wears green for fertility, her wrists tinkle with gold and green glass bangles, in her nose she wears a pearl nose ring and her face is

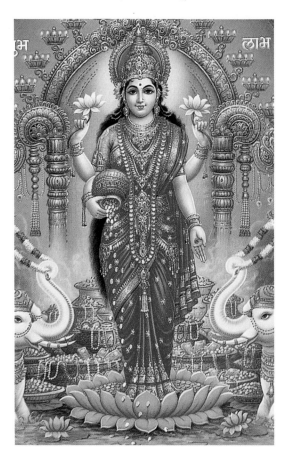

framed with strings of lustrous pearls that cascade from her temples down to her shoulders. The Gujarati bride wears red and white and has little dots of white and red drawn in an arch over her eyebrows right up to her temples.

The Indian bride is the epitome of colour and glitter. Red, fuschia, green, sunflower-yellow and saffron silks shot with threads of pure gold and silver are draped as saris and every part of the body is adorned with fabulous jewellery made of gold, pearls and precious gems. On this, her special day, she herself becomes the beautiful goddess Lakshmi, who will bring good luck and plenty to her new home and fill it with happiness and harmony.

women in the world) have been at the heart of stories of great romance and history.

Indian women have always been encouraged to make the most of their looks with cosmetics and herbs. Even in Vedic times, Sanskrit texts laid down the concept of *Sola Singaar* or the sixteen traditional accoutrements with which every woman could adorn herself. These were designed for every part of a woman's body and, irrespective of class, many of them can be fashioned out of wood, glass, fresh flowers or precious jewels.

Indian women follow the concept of *Sola Singaar* even today. While it is possible to use some of these decorations

'Her eyes are large like gentle lotuses in full bloom, her voice is as melodious as that of a singing bird in spring, her body is curved like a tender creeper encircling a tree, her silken arms are dusky like the rain filled clouds and her walk is slow and sensuous like that of a graceful elephant… she is the all-powerful goddess Parvati, who protects her devotees from every evil.' *devotional verse, sung in praise of the beautiful goddess Parvati*

sola singaar

Beautiful women have always been cherished the world over. In India too, legendary beauties such as the mythical celestial nymphs Urvashi and Menaka (who drove the gods insane with their beauty), Queen Mumtaz Mahal (in whose memory her husband Emperor Shah Jahan built the world's most magnificent tomb, the Taj Mahal) and more recently, in the mid-twentieth century, Maharani Gayatri Devi of Jaipur (rumoured at the time to be among the ten most beautiful

every day, modern life and work make others, such as armlets on the upper arm or toe rings, impractical for daily use. Many Indian women, however, even the more westernised ones, dress up in all the sixteen accoutrements for weddings, festivals and other special occasions. The sixteen accoutrements are: *bindi*, necklaces, earrings, flowers in the hair, bangles, rings, armlets on the upper arm, waistbands, anklets for the feet, kohl, toe rings, henna, perfume, sandalwood paste, the upper garment and the lower garment. They are each described below.

bindi The *bindi* is the traditional mark worn by Hindu women between the eyebrows on the forehead. It has been given different meanings at different times. It has been, and is still, seen as a sign of marriage. It has also been associated with fertility, and the red powder used to paint the dot was formerly made of a combination of mercury (considered by early Hindu alchemists to be the seed of the god Shiva, and therefore the male element), and sulphur (the female element). The practice of wearing a *bindi* is as old as the Vedas, the ancient formal texts of the Hindus that speak of the correct way of living, but today's woman still wears one, in a tradition that has lasted over 5,000 years. The *bindi* itself has, however, changed. Whereas traditional *bindi* were red, today they are worn to match with the day's outfit and come in an endless array of shapes, sizes and designs.

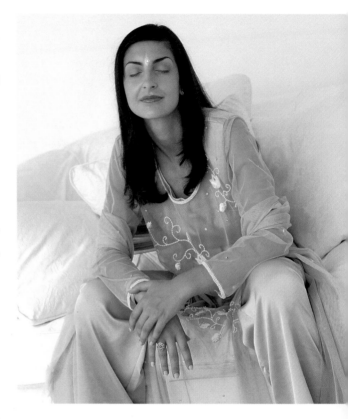

necklaces A woman highlights her best features with various pieces of jewellery. One of the most beautiful women of eighteenth-century India was Mastani, the ravishing courtesan, who captured the heart of the Maratha ruler, the Peshwa. Historians have recorded that her skin was so translucent and fragile that one could see a rosy blush stain her neck as she swallowed ruby-red pomegranate juice. She, and other beautiful maidens in Indian romantic literature, are often depicted with garlands of fresh and fragrant flowers encircling their swan-like necks. Today garlands are used as necklaces for temple deities and are also presented to special guests or newly-wed couples. Necklaces for daily wear are made of anything from gold to wood or glass.

earrings As jewellery forms an integral part of an Indian woman's attire, almost every woman has pierced ears – clip-on earrings are a western concept. In India the ears of little Hindu baby girls are ritually pierced with great ceremony on the thirteenth day after their birth. A jeweller is invited to the house and the baby's uncle (her mother's brother) holds the infant as the ears are pierced with fine gold wire that is twisted and tied into neat little loops. The family then honours the jeweller with gifts and money for decorating the daughter of the house with gold.

flowers in the hair Tiny, fragrant flowers like jasmine, *mogra*, or *saayli*, strung into chains called *gajras* are sold at every street corner. These are attached to the hair with pins or simply tucked into a plait or bun. In India no bride is completely dressed until she has a cascade of *gajras* in her hair. Even the modern Indian women will sometimes wear a *gajra* or a single colourful bloom, most often a rose, for a special, festive look.

bangles

Every married Hindu woman is called the Lakshmi, or the goddess of fortune and wealth, of her home. What she wears symbolises the financial and social status of her family. Traditionally she is expected to wear bangles, as leaving her wrists bare is inauspicious and a sign that the family has run into ill-luck.

rings

Long, slender fingers are enhanced with gold and silver rings and many Indian brides wear an ornament made of five rings, one for each finger, with little chains running from each ring to a clasped bracelet at the wrist. Hindus, Muslims and Sikhs do not traditionally wear wedding rings, although it has become fashionable since the 1980s or so to exchange engagement rings.

armlets

These are worn on the upper arm and the designs vary from region to region. One of the most popular is the snake, known for its divine powers to ward off evil and to protect stores of wealth.

waistbands

A variety of thin belts and waistbands of gold or silver, with tiny bells or motifs of gods and god-desses, are used to enhance and draw attention to the deli-cacy of womanly curves. They are usually worn with a sari which leaves the midriff bare. Broader waistbands with motifs of gods and goddesses are worn with other Indian costumes like the *ghagra* or full skirt.

anklets

Traditionally the woman of the house announces her arrival with the tinkling sound of anklets. These are always made of silver. Indians believe gold to be the metal of the gods and therefore sacred. To wear it on the feet, the lowest part of the body, is considered to be an ill-omen and disrespectful.

kohl

The eyes are the essence of appeal and allure. Black kohl is often made at home by burning a clean cotton wick in castor oil and collecting the residue of the fumes. The inner rim of the lids is then blackened with this, so that the eyes are more defined – they also benefit from the rejuvenating properties of the castor oil. It is easy to buy ready-made kohl today, but do be wary of adulterated varieties that may contain lead and will damage the eyes. Make sure that you buy reputed brands, sold by chemists and supermarkets.

toe rings

The weather in India permits women to move about barefoot. Because their feet are on show, they often decorate each toe with a different silver ring with motifs of fish, birds or flowers. In south India toe rings are a symbol of marriage and women wear a heavy ring on the second toe of each foot.

henna

The great Ayurveda practitioner Charak believed that all herbs were fathered by heaven and mothered by earth, with roots in the primeval cosmic ocean. Henna is perhaps the strongest natural colourant known to us. The dried powder of the leaves is mixed with water and the resulting paste applied

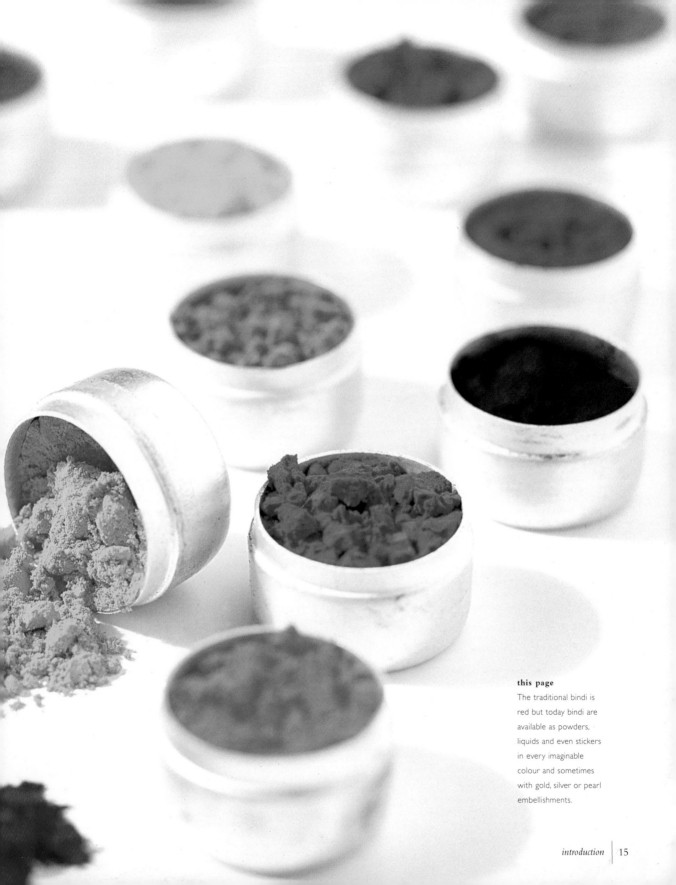

The traditional bindi is red but today bindi are available as powders, liquids and even stickers in every imaginable colour and sometimes with gold, silver or pearl embellishments.

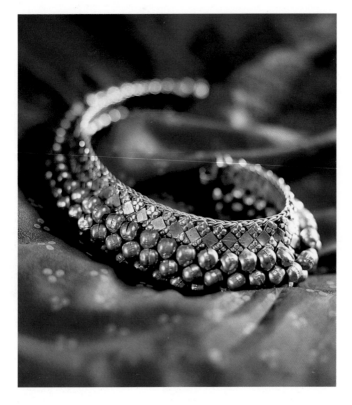

have recently discovered the pleasures of body painting and have semi-permanent tattoos painted in henna on their arms, ankles, around the navel and anywhere else they fancy. Several, including some pop stars, draw henna *bindi* on their forehead as a fashion statement.

perfume Rose, jasmine, sandalwood, lemon… these are all fragrances that are captured into *attar* or indigenously made perfume. *Attar* is available at many Indian shops in the west, although the essential oils of various fruits and flowers are more easily found at natural beauty and aromatherapy stores. *Attar* has to be used sparingly or it can become overwhelming. Most modern Indian women use commercially made perfume as it is more subtle.

above
A cluster of silver beads runs around a heavy bridal silver anklet that is too elaborate for everyday use. Many Indian women still wear light anklets every day.

to the hands, feet and hair to give a rich mahogany colour. Henna is traditionally associated with weddings and festivals, so every Indian bride will have a *mehendiwali* or henna painting artist draw filigreed patterns on her palms and feet a day before her wedding. The bride leaves the henna on overnight to dry and washes it off only the next morning before her ritual bridal bath. Friends and relatives of the bride have their hands painted with henna as well, and the day is one of great merry-making and feasting. These days henna is in demand the world over – young women

sandalwood paste One summer day when I was a teenager, my mother told me of an effective beauty secret known to generations of women in my family. 'If you want the clear, glowing skin of a queen, use sandalwood.' Every morning from then onwards I would mix together a pinch of pure sandalwood powder (made from the wood of the sandalwood tree), a pinch of turmeric (which is antiseptic), and water, and apply this to my face and neck. I am happy to say that I have never known acne and have had only the occasional pimple! Ayurveda has always recognised the cooling and polishing properties of sandalwood. Even today women apply a paste of its powder mixed with milk or water over the entire body and rinse it off when dry.

the upper garment
In Vedic times the upper garment was just a *kanchuki*, almost a strapless bra, that covered the breasts and could be made of cloth or tree bark. Nowadays the upper garment has come to mean the blouse worn with a sari.

the lower garment
About five hundred years ago the lower garment was a cloth held up at the waist with a string or belt. Today it is synonymous with the sari, which is worn in innumerable ways. The most popular is the five-yard sari, an unstitched length of cloth, one end of which is pleated in front and the other end thrown over the left shoulder. Saris are made of silk, cotton or synthetic fabrics and the best ones are woven by hand at various weaving centres all over India. According to legend, the weaver who made the first sari captured in his creation all that he thought symbolised woman. He translated her softness into the texture, her strength into its tenacity, the beauty of her smile into the sparkling colour and her tears into its rippling cascade.

below
According to Ayurveda both sandalwood and henna are cooling, and are therefore used especially in the long, hot summer months. Henna gives colour whereas sandalwood smooths and perfumes the skin.

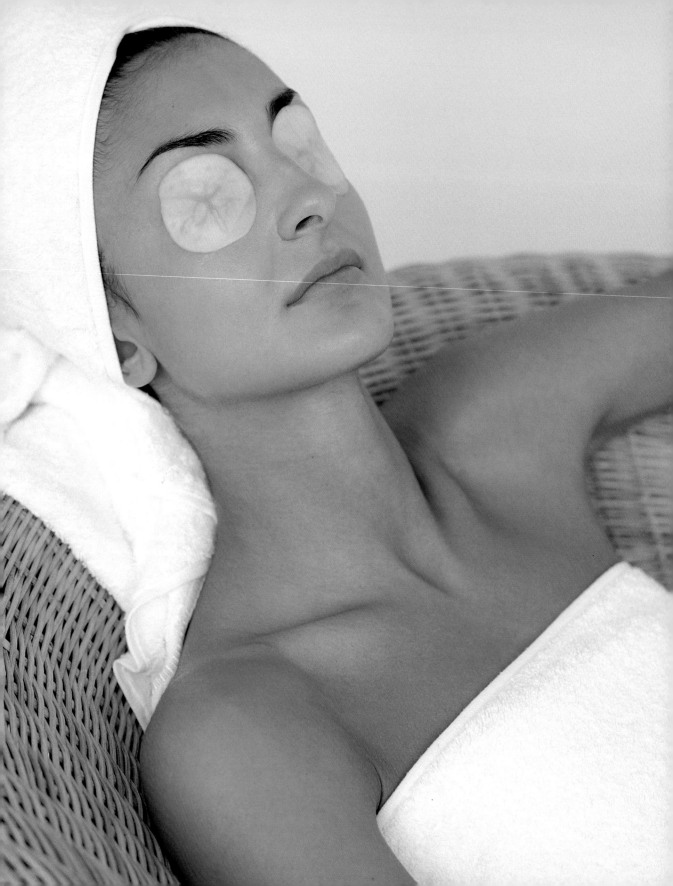

'The flowery arrows of her veiled gaze pierced the haven of his heart;
Their eyes slowly met and set their love ablaze.' *Urdu love song*

eyes & lashes

The allure of the eyes is beautifully expressed in a popular story where a young Lord Krishna asks his mother Yashodha why he is so dark-skinned while his lady love Radha is so fair. Yashodha laughs and replies, 'Lovely Radha's eyes are lined with dark kohl and those dark, sparkling eyes have mesmerised you, my son – that is why you are so dark.' Health and happiness first radiate through the eyes. Indian women are known for their large, lustrous eyes.

The first step towards lovely eyes is to eliminate strain. Strained eyes look red and puffy and are often surrounded by tiny wrinkles popularly known as crow's feet. An effective way to soothe eyestrain is to place cotton pads soaked in cool rosewater (which has been recommended by Indian herbalists for centuries because of its cooling properties) on the closed eyelids for 10–15 minutes. Better still, warm, used tea bags make an excellent reviver for tired eyes as the tannin in the tea is a stimulant and gives instant sparkle. Another good reviver for dull eyes readily available from chemists' shops in the west is a compress of witch-hazel, a liquid made from the extract of the bark and leaves of the tree of the same name, which grows most abundantly in North America. It also grows in India and Ayurveda mentions it for its refreshing and stimulating properties. Lie down with a cotton pad soaked in witch-hazel on each closed eye for ten minutes to feel completely relaxed. Soft music and dim lights will further help to relieve stress.

Ayurveda tells us that we are what we eat. Drinking plenty of water through the day flushes out toxins and keeps the eyes clear and healthy. A good diet with plenty of vitamins A and C found in green and yellow fruits and vegetables, along with proteins found in meat, fish and dairy foods, helps to keep the eyes healthy and bright.

Needless to say, the golden rule for healthy sparkling eyes is to have adequate sleep and fresh air. Also, all Indian women know that it is unwise to step out in the hot, tropical afternoon sun when the eyes naturally squint to focus in the bright light. Modern women who work outdoors never go without a good pair of sunglasses. My grandmother Uma would always tell me when I was a schoolgirl that the hot sun was poison for the eyes and for the complexion, warning, 'Don't play in the sun or you will bake till you are like bark and you will grow up squinting like a bad-tempered old woman.'

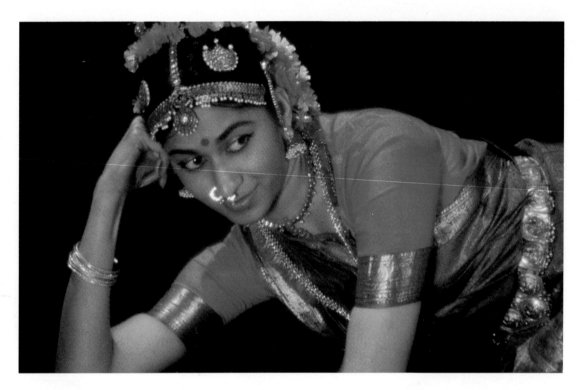

above

A classical Indian dancer
can tell entire stories
through her eyes. Here a
lovelorn heroine awaits
the arrival of her truant
lover, her impatient gaze
fixed on the winding path
that leads to her home.

lashes

'I am smitten with love as you gaze at me through the dark, velvety curtain of your lashes,' sings the hero to the beautiful heroine of many a Hindi film. Which woman has not longed for a fringe of thick, dark lashes to frame her eyes? Long eyelashes are prized in every culture and are quite easy to achieve through very simple routines. It is well known that natural beauty treatments are repaid with glorious good looks that need little or no help from make-up.

According to Ayurveda, castor oil is the most cooling of oils. Excessive body heat hampers the growth of hair. A tiny smear of castor oil on the lashes at bedtime is known to thicken them. In India even little girls' eyes are decorated with kohl or *kajal* that has castor oil which helps eyelashes grow thick and strong. Remember too that eyelashes, like the hair on all the other parts of the body, have a growth cycle. They grow, rest and fall out, to be replaced by new hair in a few weeks. The life span of each lash is about five months and, in most circumstances, sparse eyelashes will be a temporary phase. Leaving mascara on overnight clogs the follicles, so remove all make up before sleeping.

dark circles

Dark circles can be hereditary or can appear as a result of illness or lack of sleep. Anaemia, excessive tiredness or heavy periods can also be the cause, as can a considerable reduction in fluid intake if you are on a crash diet. Some Western women acquire dark circles in old age. A well-known actress in Indian films is reputed to have shadowy dark circles as part of her natural complexion. She has tried in vain to eliminate them and now depends entirely on good make-up tricks for her flawless skin tone. It is sometimes impossible to erase what nature has given us, although nature also provides some of the most valuable answers to our problems. Slices of potato or even a potato compress placed on closed eyelids go a long way in reducing dark circles. To make a potato compress, just grate a small, raw potato and fill into two thin cloth pouches. Keep these over your lids for 15–20 minutes every other day. The starch in the potatoes 'lifts' the skin, helping to fade dark circles gradually. If your lids feel a little dry after this treatment, just apply a smear of almond or olive oil before going to bed. Apples also make a fragrant eye pad, as they are rich in assimilable minerals such as potassium, vitamins B and C, and tannin, all of which assist in eliminating dark circles. A slice on each eye for ten minutes or so will do wonders.

puffiness

Dark circles are often accompanied by puffiness or 'bags' under the eyes. Some of this may be due to poor circulation or particular allergies and the use of rich night creams. The skin under the eyes is extremely delicate and allows oil or cream to seep in and stay there. Avoid using rich creams around the eyes for long periods of time. Puffiness on waking in the morning could be due to fluid retention in the tissues, which some beauticians believe is due to lack of blinking at night. Drink a glass of hot water in bed (keep a vacuum flask on your beside table) as soon as you wake up, and lie back for another ten minutes. According to Ayurvedic doctors, the water kick-starts the kidneys, which have slowed down during sleep, into working normally again, thus drawing out retained water from the tissues.

The instant, but temporary, Indian home remedy for puffy eyes is to apply a compress of a weak solution of sea-salt and water. The salt draws water away from the tissues and leaves the eyes looking fresh. You must rinse the eyes with cool water immediately afterwards to remove all traces of salt, which might sting.

fine lines & wrinkles

Fine lines appear around the eyes as we age, though they may be worsened by excessive dryness of the skin, squinting – and laughter. The skin around the eyes is very delicate and a light smear of pure almond oil (or olive oil, which is more easily available) twenty minutes before bedtime helps to soften dry skin. Wipe off gently with moist cottonwool before sleeping so that it does not give you puffy eyes the next morning. Many of India's leading herbal beauticians also believe that a very light daily application of a good, natural anti-wrinkle solution like witch-hazel around the eyes delays the onset of crow's feet and can even ease out some of the early ones if they have already appeared.

Do use cautiously: if witch-hazel gets into the
eyes it can smart quite painfully. The following
recipes, which have been collected from family
and friends, have been tried and tested for
many years. They take into account that
certain ingredients will be available only
during certain seasons.

Smita's eye-wash for hot eyes

My friend Smita gave me this recipe for an
eye-wash that cools tired or sunburnt eyes –
'hot eyes' as she calls the condition.

½ tsp **green fennel seeds**
½ tsp **coriander seeds**
A slice of a fresh, purple fig

Put all the ingredients into a pan with a cup of
water and bring to the boil. Lower the heat
and simmer for five minutes. Strain well, cool
and use as an eye-wash. This is done by filling a
small clean eye-cup, which fits neatly over the
eye, with the wash. Bend your head forward to
place one eye over the cup snugly, then tilt
head back and let the liquid bathe the eye well.
Repeat the procedure for the other eye after
cleaning the cup and filling it with fresh fluid.

It is well known in India that Ayurveda
recommends both fennel and coriander for

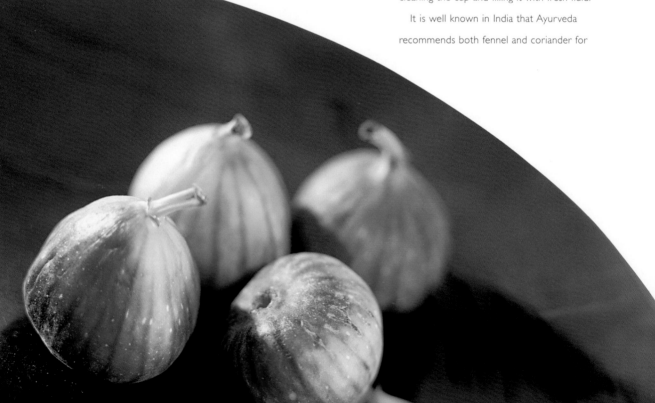

their cooling properties. These spices help to draw heat away from the eyes and therefore improve vision. Purple figs are an extremely rich source of Vitamin A, the 'eye' vitamin, and are said to rejuvenate tired eyes.

Malti's under-eye remedy for dark circles

My aunt Malti swears by the juice of mint although she can't explain exactly how it helps. The almond oil has gentle lubricating properties, which help to dispel fine lines and dark patches due to dry skin. Honey is an ideal energizing food and according to Ayurveda has a tremendous healing effect on the body.

5 fresh mint leaves

1 tsp almond oil

½ tsp honey

Crush the mint with a little water in a mortar. Strain the juice and add to the almond oil and honey. Stir till completely mixed and apply a tiny amount under the eyes before going to bed.

exercises to improve vision

Ancient Indian yogis and practitioners of yoga always included eye exercises in their daily routine so as to keep the 'windows to the soul', as well as perhaps the most important of

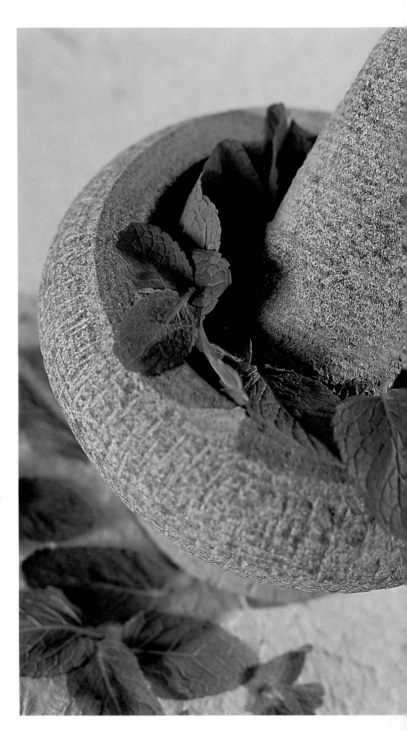

the senses, alive and healthy. Even today ophthalmic experts all over the world. recommend yogic exercises. The following exercises relieve tired eyes, help to improve vision and reduce fine lines and 'bags' under the eyes.

1 The simplest exercise is rapid blinking. We usually blink once every four seconds, but making an effort to blink in quick succession about ten times eases tiredness immediately. You can repeat this exercise up to five times a day.

2 Another basic exercise is to scrunch the eyelids together as tightly as you can for just a second and then relax them again. Gently iron out the delicate skin under the eyes with the pad of your little finger to stop fine lines from forming – never apply pressure to the eyes or the skin around them. Do this exercise three times daily.

3 Rolling the eyes without moving the head is an effective exercise to motivate sluggish eye muscles to work better. Do this three times in each direction, starting by rolling the eyes upwards and going all the way round.

4 Do the same as in the preceding exercise, but imagine that you are drawing a square with your eyes. Keep the square as big as possible and do not cut any corners. Palming is an effective way of relaxing the eyes.

5 Extend your right arm in front of you. Swing it very slowly horizontally till it is in line with your shoulder and beyond. Follow the arm with your eyes without moving your head. Continue as far as your vision keeps up with your arm, then bring the arm and your eyes slowly back to the front. Repeat with the left arm. Do this exercise once daily.

6 Simply lean your elbows on a table, cup your palms and place them over your eyes. Blink a few times, then shut your eyes and relax the eyes and. face. Sit still for about five minutes, then open your eyes and remove your hands. Be careful not to place pressure on your eyes at any point. You can do this any number of times each day. It is particularly useful if you work in a visually challenging job, such as with computers.

7 Lift your eyes to the ceiling diagonally and across to the floor on the opposite side. Lift to the ceiling again and diagonally across to the floor in the opposite direction. Repeat this exercise five times.

8 Help your eyes to adjust to a change in focus with this exercise. Look intently at a distant object, then quickly bring your gaze to something at arm's length. Repeat this exercise five times. This exercise is discreet enough to do while travelling or at work.

9 According to yoga, one of the best exercises for improving vision is the practice of *shirshasan* or balancing upside-down on the head. You can use the support of a wall to keep the back straight. The rush of blood to the head promotes circulation around the eyes

right
Always keep your eye make-up in mint condition. Old, dusty pencils can be an ideal breeding ground for fungus and can give you an eye infection. Replace your make-up every 3–6 months.

and therefore helps vision. For those who are a little faint-hearted, sit on a chair with the head dropped down between the knees. Try to reach for the floor with the crown of your head. Hold this position for five minutes and do it once a week to begin with.

10 Shut your eyes. With the ring finger of each hand gently massage the eyelids and through them the eyeballs, using small circular movements. Do this for 2–3 minutes.

make-up

'Her eyes are electrifying like a bird's wings in flight' and 'her eyes dance like bees', are just two of the descriptions of the beautiful goddess Parvati in the sacred Hindu hymn the *Shivalilamrit*. The most beautiful eyes in the world have a mysterious sparkle and a secret allure that touch the eyes of the beholder. Whatever the shape and size of the eyes we possess, we all aspire to evenly shaped, well-defined eyes that are framed with a fringe of thick lashes. Make-up was created so that we could improve on nature and give ourselves the look we dream about. In India large, almond-shaped eyes are prized and women use all sorts of eye make-up to create this illusion.

eyebrows

The majority of Indian women shape their eyebrows to create an archway to the eyes. The most common method of doing this is 'threading',

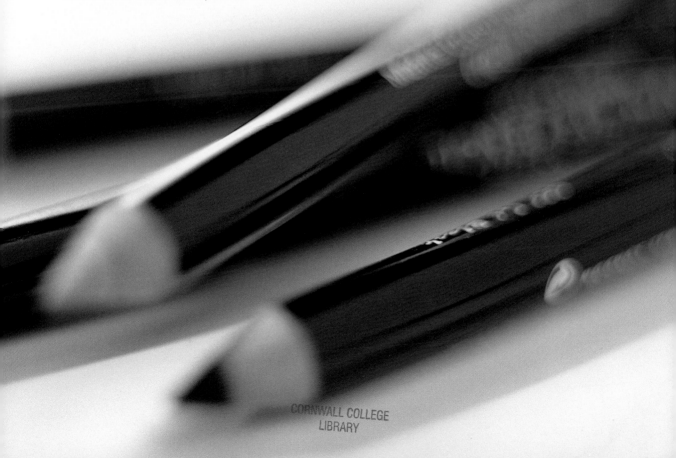

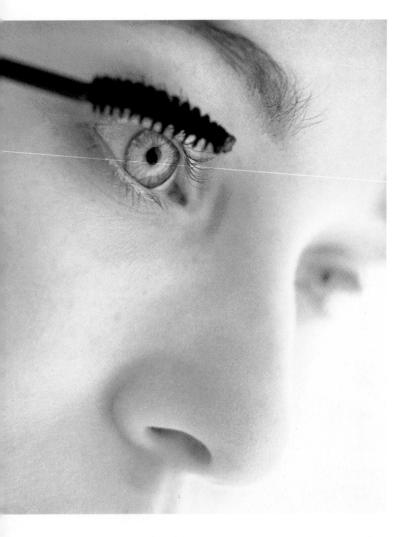

Here is a trick that grandmother taught us to determine the correct length for our eyebrows. Hold a pencil against the outside of your nostril and align it to the inner corner of your eye. The top of the pencil will point to where your eyebrows should begin. Gradually shift the top of the pencil across the eye till it is perpendicular to the nose and aligns with the outer corner of the eye. The tip of the pencil will now point to where the eyebrow should end. If your eyebrows are sparse, fill any gaps with light, feathery strokes of a sharp but soft pencil, a colour that matches your eyebrows. Always brush your eyebrows upwards and outwards after making up your face.

shadow, eyeliner, mascara & kohl
Although fashions change, certain shading tricks to enhance the shape of the eyes can be used at all times. For eyes that are close set, for example, lighter-coloured eyeshadow should be used on the inner portion of the lid towards the nose and darker eyeshadow on the outer edge of the lid. Reverse this technique for widely space eyes.

Every year in October, Hindus celebrate the festival of Navratri, in honour of the fiery goddess Durga who, according to legend, fought the evil demon Mahishasura for nine days and nine nights, eventually to slay him and save the world. Sculptors make flamboyant clay images and masks of this beautiful

above
Mascara instantly 'opens' the eyes and adds to feminine allure. Coat the lashes evenly keeping your gaze as steady as possible to avoid smudging. For the same reasons, don't overload the wand with mascara.

where ordinary cotton thread is manipulated within the fingers of both hands to pluck out unwanted or stray hairs until a neat crescent shape is achieved (see page 94). Of course you can use tweezers if you prefer. Shaping the eyebrows instantly tidies up the face and focuses attention on the eyes.

goddess, who rides a lion. Her eyes are shown to be her most enchanting feature and artists draw attention to them by outlining both lids with black eyeliner. The liner is gently flicked out and upwards at the outer edge of each eye. The inner rim of the lower lid is lined with kohl and the lashes are coated in dark mascara. The magnetism of those eyes draws devotees to her like moths to a bright flame.

Eyeliner must be used with care if it is to have the desire result. Liquid liner can look harsh as it does not blend or diffuse; a soft but sharp pencil is easier to use, and neutral, smoky colours such as brown, grey or charcoal are the most natural. The pencil line can be smudged for a softer look. Evening make-up is heavier than that worn during the day – build up on the colour and add gold or silver for intensity and drama.

Every pair of feminine eyes in the world looks better with a coat of mascara. Mascara not only makes the lashes seem thicker but also darkens them and adds to their length. The best way to apply it is in several thin coats, separating the lashes as you go along and avoiding unsightly clumps. Coat the top of the upper lashes in neat strokes, then their underside. Repeat for the lower lashes. All this takes time, but is well worth the effort.

Remember, never allow yourself to go to sleep without removing your make-up. The eyes and surrounding area are extremely sensitive and any neglect or lack of care will show up immediately. Remove all make-up gently but thoroughly with eye make-up remover or pure oil (coconut or almond is good). Wipe off gently with a swab of moist cotton wool and rinse off all the oil before going to bed.

communicating with your eyes

The first form of communication between a mother and her newborn baby is through the eyes. Best friends speak volumes to each other with just a look and lovers can touch each other secretly with meaningful glances.

If you remember the moment you fell in love or met the person of your dreams, you will recall the message that passed between the eyes – interest, question, reciprocation, joy, excitement… The eyes start the story of romance and intensify it. Be careful of the signals you send out and the effect they may have. According to the *Kamasutra*, 'a girl shows her love by outward signs and actions… she never looks at the man in the face, she looks secretly at him though he has gone away from her side…'

In the Hindu marriage ceremony a groom shows his bride the Pole Star (the steadfast star seen in the northern part of the sky) with the words, 'Firm art thou; I see thee, the firm one. Firm be thou with me, O thriving one! To me

'a girl shows her love by outward signs and actions, such as the following, she never looks at the man in the face, she looks secretly at him though he has gone away from her side…' *Kamasutra*

Brihaspati has given thee, obtaining offsprings through me, thy husband, live with me a hundred autumns.' These words are taken from the *Gruha Sutras*, which are a part of the Vedas and lay down the procedure for rituals and sacraments. The bride is expected to be steady of eye, heart and soul like the unflickering Pole star and thus strengthen the bond of conjugal life.

Even in business, maintaining eye contact is crucial and can often be your strongest ally in closing a deal.

'Mother, the ocean of love in your eyes, envelopes me through the war of life.' *Prayer to Parvati*

According to a Hindu legend, Lord Shiva was unwittingly disturbed in his penance by the god of love, Kama, who mistook him for a deer. The closed third eye of Shiva, located in his forehead, flashed open and reduced Kama to ashes with a single bolt of lightning. This story illustrates the power and energy that is attributed to the eyes. Even today Indians believe that a positive, well-meaning soul is reflected in clear, focused eyes.

In situations where you feel flustered or anxious don't allow your eyes to flit around (this can be most off-putting), take a few deep breaths and try to organise your thoughts . Another easy way to appear in control while talking to someone is to shift your focus to someone or something else in the room for a minute or so, keeping the gaze steady all the time. This will camouflage your nervousness while giving you a chance to collect your thoughts.

yogic exercises to intensify the gaze

Try this simple exercise. Look at the tip of your nose for a minute, then focus on an object far away for another minute. Choose a different object each time. Do this for five minutes every day until the eyes develop an unwavering gaze.

One of the most powerful lessons of *hatha-yoga* (a physical doctrine to elevate the spiritual) for increasing the intensity of the gaze is *tratak sadhana*. This exercise has been practised by yogis and spiritual people for thousands of years. Yoga itself is one of the six orthodox systems of Hindu philosophy and there is evidence to show that it was practised in some form during the Indus Valley Civilisation of around 2500–1500 BC. The purpose of *tratak sadhana* is to focus one's energy through the eyes and to develop extra-sensory perception and mind power. Once you have achieved some mastery over this *sadhana*, your eyes will be able to communicate your thoughts much more powerfully.

Here is what to do: sit in front of a mirror (for some reason the best time to do this is at dusk), in a comfortable but erect position, focus your eyes, and therefore your mind, on an imaginary spot between your eyebrows and concentrate. Learn to concentrate your energy into this spot until you can see nothing else. Yoga advises that *tratak sadhana* should be practised every day. Start with a couple of minutes and increase the time as you go along.

right
A mother and her baby constantly talk to each through their eyes. Happy, smiling eyes give a feeling of warmth and security whereas a stern look is enough to make a baby cry.

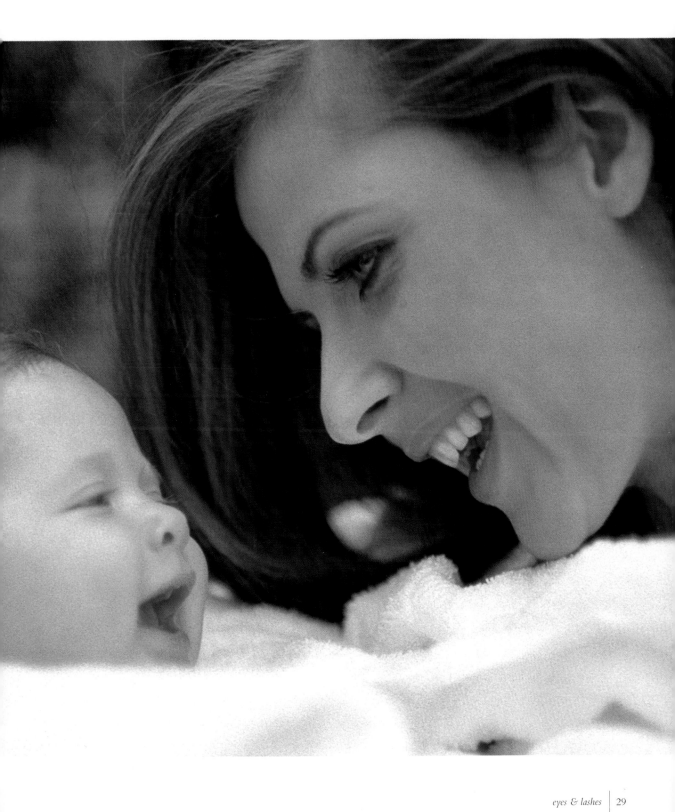

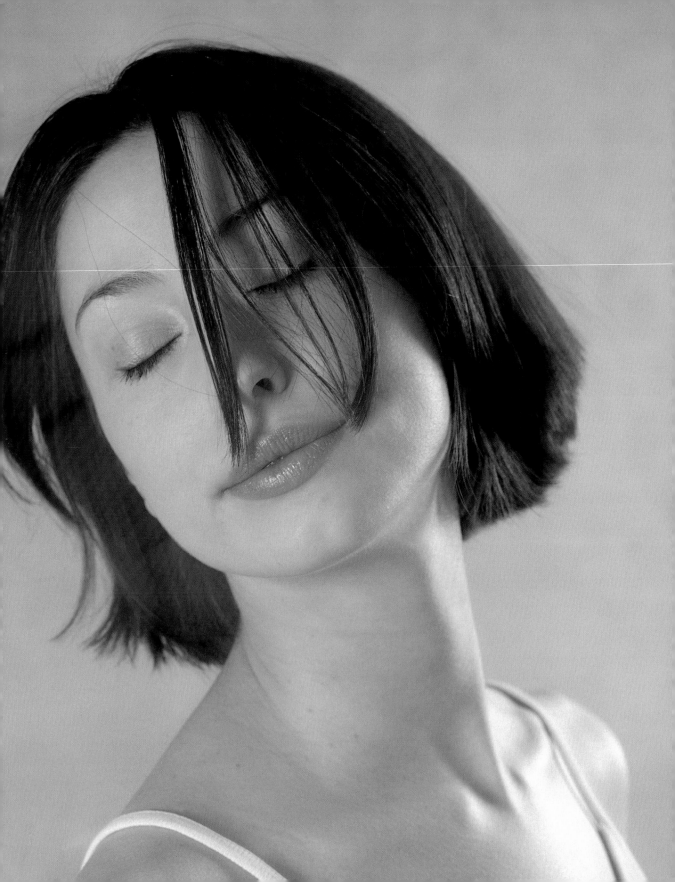

'Dawn comes on the waves of pink and gold cloud

Her richly ornamented face brings joy to the world

With a radiant face this daughter of heaven looks glorious

Her splendid face shows wisdom, divine beauty,

As she comes escorted by the sun's rays.'

hymn to Ushas, the goddess of dawn, from the Rigveda

face & neck

Although your skin accounts for only a tenth of your body weight, it is the complexion of your face and neck that is seen and noticed first. In fact, all through the winter the only two areas 'on show' are your face and neck, whereas the summer heralds a more liberal display of the skin.

One of the prerequisites of beauty is healthy, smooth skin. Every woman strives for a flawless complexion and in India girls traditionally start looking after the skin on their face and neck from an early age. Natural kitchen ingredients are easily available and mother is always nearby to give advice and support. Starting early ensures that by the thirties, when fine lines normally appear or the skin loses some of its elasticity, it is already well prepared. Today, with the extra onslaught of pollution, stress, bad eating habits and the lack of time for proper skin care, it is all the more vital that we develop routines that will keep the face and neck looking radiant and youthful for as long as possible.

Even the sages who lived in India during the Vedic period knew that two of the most important treatments for the skin were fresh air and water.

air

Although the skin receives most of its supply of oxygen from the bloodstream, it takes in up to 2.5 percent of the body's total oxygen requirement by direct absorption from the environment. The skin also directly expels about 3 percent of the body's carbon dioxide waste. This ability of the skin has led beauticians across the world to advise women to let their skin 'breathe'. A clean skin is also a vehicle for the free exchange of moisture. There is no doubt that if this function of the skin is hampered and the toxins produced by the body are trapped in the skin, the quality and health of the skin will suffer.

Nonetheless, most women, especially in the West, are encouraged to cover their skin at all times. During the day, moisturisers and lotions are layered on to the face, some of which create an occlusive film that prevents the natural exchange of gases through the skin. At night, richer creams are prescribed to combat the day's ravages. Scientists have proved, however, that most absorption takes place within the first twenty minutes or so: after that the cream acts only as a barrier for air. It is better to wipe off any cream after twenty minutes and leave the face bare throughout the night. Alternatively, you could use a lighter moisturiser. A daily walk in fresh air, however cold the weather, will also improve circulation and give the skin a glow. Take care, though, of strong sun or wind as these will only speed up the signs of ageing.

water

The best toner for your skin is ice-cold water. Women who live in the Himalayan mountains in the northernmost part of India cleanse their faces with water from mountain streams that are fed by snowy glaciers throughout the year. No wonder, then, that their complexions glow with health and vigour! Icy water stimulates the cells, perks up circulation and helps to close open pores. It is instantly refreshing and I like to splash it on after applying foundation to set my make-up and keep it looking fresh till I want to take it off. In very hot weather I tie an ice cube in a piece of muslin and rub it on my face, two to three times a day, to eliminate excess oil on the nose or forehead and to cool the skin. Beauticians advise against using ice directly on the skin as this may lead to burst capillaries which form ugly red patches under the skin. One of the best pick-me-ups for your skin is to wash the face and neck with cold water first thing in the morning until it tingles and feels 'wide awake' – it's also a great way to get you going!

your emotions

All of us know that when we are sad or depressed, the skin feels and looks mottled and pasty. The skin is a mirror for what we are feeling and will show dark circles, uneven patches and blemishes within a matter of a few hours.

According to the *Yog-Sutra* of Patanjali, probably written around AD 200, steadfastness of mind and detachment from pain or pleasure help us rise above the daily grind of the world: 'By meditation upon light and upon radiance, knowledge of the spirit can be reached and therefore peace can be achieved.' Here 'light and radiance' refer to good thoughts and the positive energy that is found in everyone and everywhere. All Hindu scriptures speak of keeping the mind steady so that emotions cannot toss you about like a ship in troubled waters. It pays to follows this advice, not least for the sake of your looks. Anger and tension not only upset your equilibrium but also activate your sebaceous glands to produce excess oil, which in turn leads to rashes, spots and blotches.

types of skin

Healthy skin glows with radiance and is smooth and soft. Whatever your skin type – oily, combination or dry – you can encourage it to its best possible state with regular care and perseverance.

oily skin

Oily skin is a result of over-active sebaceous glands. It shines in patches, is prone to spots and does not hold on to make-up for long. It comes with enlarged pores and an oily scalp, but the good news is that it will develop fewer wrinkles and maintains its elasticity and youthfulness longer.

The most important routine for oily skin is cleansing. You will notice that water-based cleansers work best and a good herbal soap and water are the simplest and most effective. In India women make a paste of *multani mitti* or fuller's earth (available at most Indian shops in the West) and water and apply this as a face and neck mask twice a week to cleanse and smooth oily skin. A mask of oatmeal and almond powder mixed with water is an excellent substitute. Once a week apply a well-beaten mixture of egg white and a few drops of lemon juice to your face and neck to tighten the skin and close the pores. Be sure to use all your masks as soon as you have made them up as they will not keep.

dry skin

Dry skin has a matt texture, tends to flake and looks white or grey in patches. Often dry skin is aggravated because the sebaceous glands are lazy or the skin has been over-exposed to the harsh elements – wind, sun or sea. Central heating also worsens dry skin. Unfortunately, in this type of skin, wrinkles develop early and dryness tends to intensify with age.

Even dry skin needs a good cleanser. Use oil (baby oil is the gentlest) to wipe off make-up and grime. Avoid all astringents, but do

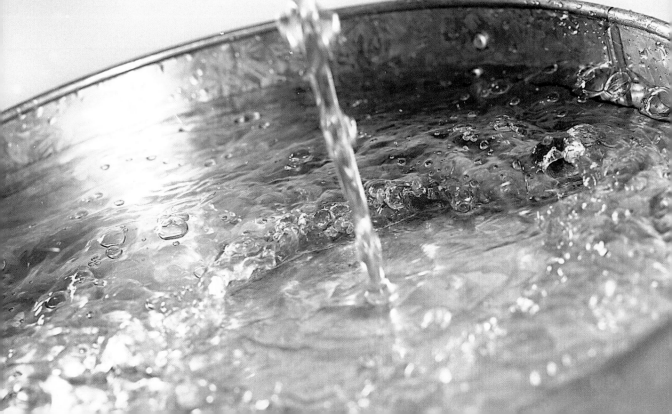

below

Summer is an ideal season to refresh your skin with a cube of luscious, fragrant, golden melon. Dry skin especially benefits from a juicy but gentle massage

moisturise often and as thoroughly as possible. Leave the moisturiser on the skin as a protective film. Dry skin appreciates a weekly face mask that is nourishing and rejuvenating. Gently scrub off dead skin with a teaspoonful of oatmeal or, better still, chickpea flour which is used all over India and is known for its softening properties. Then mix together an egg yolk with a teaspoonful of honey and spread over the face and neck. Leave for twenty minutes, then rinse off. When I was a girl, my grandmother Uma would often give me a cube of cool melon to rub on my face. She said that the juice would make even my dry skin glow. For some reason it did, and I loved the fresh smell that lingered around me for hours afterwards. Another little trick of hers was to apply a smear of almond oil to my face after a bath while my skin was still damp. That tightly-pulled discomfort of dry skin magically disappeared.

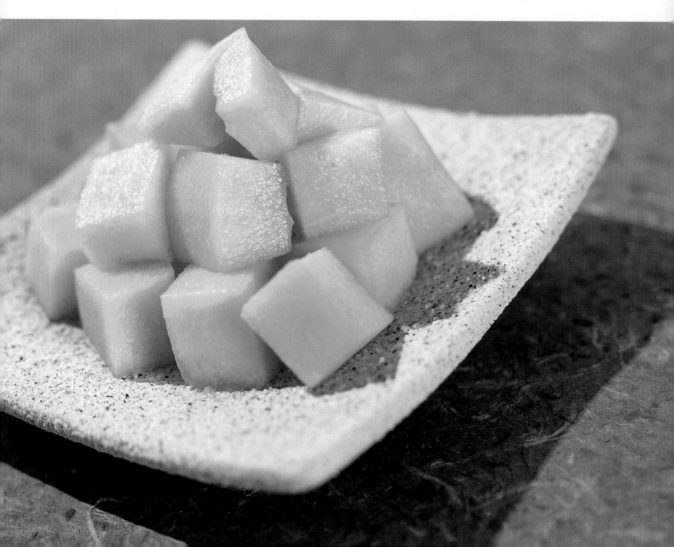

combination skin

Combination skin has dry and oily areas. The oily areas classically form a T-shape over the face to include the forehead, nose and chin, while the skin around the eyes tends to be dry.

It is impractical to use different types of products for different areas of the face, so just use more or less of the same product – moisturise the dry areas a little more richly than the oily ones and cleanse the oily ones more deeply. Use a light under-eye cream every other night. My friend Gita tells me that her mother created a home-made mask of fresh parsley juice (just crush the leaves with a pestle and mortar) and honey that was guaranteed to even out combination skin. She remembers walking around the house with a bright green face and scampering into one of the inner rooms of their large, leafy bungalow when any unexpected visitors arrived.

Yoghurt is an essential part of the Indian diet – we eat it with rice, rotis (wholewheat Indian bread), in sweets and on its own with salt or sugar, and consider it, as confirmed by Ayurveda, to be one of nature's most equalising foods. Use it (preferably live or bio-yoghurt) on your face to 'neutralise' combination skin. A maximum of twenty minutes once a week is more than enough.

normal skin

Draupadi, the heroine of the epic *Mahabharata*, was also known as 'Yagyaseni' or 'born of fire' because, according to legend, she was created from a sacred fire. Draupadi is considered to be one of the five most beautiful women of Indian mythology – her skin was burnished gold and smooth as the softest silk. The lustre of her perfect, fire-glowing skin was known far and wide, and in her time she was the most sought-after woman in India.

You are truly blessed if you have smooth, unblemished skin with no enlarged pores. Even so, normal skin still needs looking after. Regular cleansing, toning and moisturising will pay rich dividends in maintaining the quality of the skin. A facial a fortnight keeps it glowing. Normal skin benefits from a variety of kitchen ingredients. Rub a piece of any ripe, slightly acidic soft fruit (Indian women use mango, grape or guava, but you can substitute a strawberry or raspberry) on your face and neck to boost the circulation and enliven the skin. The fruit acids work in many ways: they mildly exfoliate, rejuvenate, tone and soften the skin within minutes and envelop you in an aura of delicious fragrance.

three steps to beautiful skin

There are three daily steps to a beautiful skin whatever its type: cleansing to remove grime, excess oil and make-up; toning to close pores, refine and rejuvenate; and moisturising to hydrate and keep it supple. Moisturisers work by sealing water into the skin and preventing it from being evaporated from the skin cells. Even the best skin needs a good moisturiser.

Here are a few recipes and techniques for you to try at home. They are all fun and easy to make or do and have been used by Indian women for many hundreds of years. Always prepare only small quantities of any recipe, so that you can use it up quickly. Home recipes do not contain any preservatives (unlike commercial products) and can be breeding grounds for bacteria if stored for too long or in the wrong conditions.

cleansers

cleansing face mask

The oatmeal in this mask sloughs off dead surface skin and the buttermilk or whey, which is mildly acidic, reaches deep into the pores to clean dirt and grime. Also, buttermilk contains all the casein (protein) and the mineral salts found in milk, which nourish the skin while cleansing.

2 tbsp oatmeal

about 4 tbsp buttermilk or whey (see method)

To make buttermilk, blend full-fat set plain live yoghurt with a few spoons of ice-cold water till the butterfat separates from the liquid, this liquid is buttermilk. If buttermilk is difficult to make or buy, whey – the water that appears on top of set plain live yoghurt on keeping – works just as well.

Mix the oatmeal with the buttermilk or whey to form a smooth paste. Apply this paste all over the face and neck and leave on for ten to fifteen minutes. Rinse off with cool water and pat dry. This mask can be used once a week on any skin type.

exfoliating scrub for normal skin

6 almonds

milk to mix

Soak the almonds in the milk overnight. Blend together coarsely the next morning and use all over the face in gentle circular motions. Leave for five minutes, then rinse off with cool water.

steaming An effective method of deep-cleansing the skin, used by many Indian women, is steaming. It opens the pores so that they can be emptied of oil and dirt more effectively. Never steam your face over boiling water on a stove – it could scald your skin. Take the pan off the stove, make a tent over your head with a thick towel and let your face

far right
Oatmeal is ideal for a face mask – it cleanses away dull or dead skin to give a fresh glow to your face.

below
Perfectly natural seaweed soap preserves the natural oil in your skin while beautifully cleansing it with its rich lather.

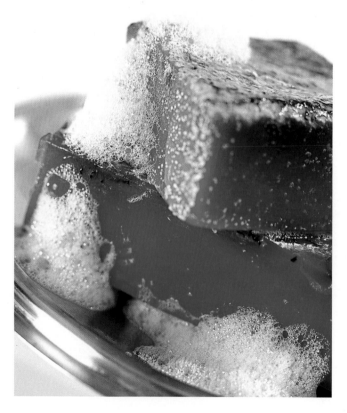

luxuriate in the warmth of the steam for about seven to ten minutes. Although plain water works wonderfully, adding a handful of herbs or flowers adds extra dash. Jasmine flowers have anti-bacterial properties and add a delightful fragrance that is mildly aphrodisiac. Basil leaves are antiseptic and clear skin blemishes. Take care not to over-steam the face as this can encourage the development of permanently open pores. Once a month should be more than enough.

toners

a very simple skin tonic

Grapes have a very high-quality sugar content as well as enzymes that smooth and refine the skin.

a couple of large, juicy grapes

Split the grapes in half and rub over the face and neck. Leave for half an hour and rinse off.

a natural toner

One of the best toners you can use is mineral water. Just empty some into a natural spray container and fizz your face from time to time to set make-up, tone the skin or to revive and refresh yourself instantly.

Mala's toner for oily skin

1 cup finely grated raw cabbage

2 tsp rosewater

Put the grated cabbage in a muslin square and squeeze out the juice. Mix this with the rosewater and pat on to the face and neck. Allow to dry, then rinse off.

moisturisers

Moisturising forms an even more important part of
your beauty routine during the winter months. Always
remember to treat your neck to all the goodies you use
on your face – otherwise you will end up with a lovely face
on a crepey neck!

night cream

The cocoa in this moisturiser will not stain the face.
Instead the alkaloids it contains – mainly theobromine and
caffeine – act as stimulants and rejuvenate the skin. Lanolin
is available from health and specialist beauty shops.

2 tbsp almond oil

2 tbsp lanolin

1 tsp cocoa powder

2 tbsp rosewater

Put the almond oil, lanolin and cocoa in a heatproof glass
bowl. Place the bowl over a pan of water and heat gently
over a low heat till the mixture melts into a smooth cream.
Use only a wooden spoon to stir as a metal one will react
with the ingredients. Take off the heat and add the rosewater, stirring all the while. Allow the cream to cool and store
in a glass bottle.

liquorice moisturising cream

Liquorice is one of the most powerful herbs of the
Oriental Materia Medica and Ayurveda suggests its use as
a skin nourisher and to give the skin luminiscence. It is
available from herbalists and health shops. Do scrape off the
outer skin of the root before infusing it in water as this
does not have the good qualities of the root within.

1 tsp liquorice root

2 tbsp almond oil

1 tbsp bees wax

Steep the liquorice root in 3 tbsp water for 6 hours. Put
the beeswax and oil into a heatproof glass bowl, place over
a pan of hot water and melt over a low heat. Remove from
the heat and beat in the strained liquorice infusion. Keep
stirring till the cream cools and thickens.

face masks

The most luxurious beauty treatment for the face is
the application of a face pack. It deep-cleans, tones and
moisturises all at once, smells delicious and makes you feel
relaxed and pampered. Face masks are simple to make and
can easily save you money spent on commercial products.

for an oily skin

Sandalwood is a natural astringent. Turmeric is antiseptic
and keeps spots in check, while the fruit acid in orange
juice clears blemishes. The turmeric may stain the skin
slightly, but this is temporary and will clear after a few
washes. If you have sensitive skin and are worried about
staining, substitute the turmeric with geranium leaf juice
(crush one leaf with a little water, strain and use ½ tsp of
the liquid), reducing the quantity of orange juice by the
same amount.

1½ tbsp sandalwood powder

tiny pinch (few grains) of ground turmeric

3 tbsp orange juice

Mix all the ingredients together and apply over the face and neck, avoiding the eye area. Allow to dry, then rinse off with cool water, without pulling the skin.

for dry skin

This mask conditions dry skin and leaves it supple and radiant.

1 egg white

1 tsp honey

1 tsp full-fat cream

Mix together all the ingredients and pat on to the face and neck. Rinse off after 20 minutes.

for normal skin

The protein in milk powder leaves skin petal-soft and the rosewater tones and refreshes.

2 tbsp milk powder

rosewater to mix

Combine the ingredients into a thick paste and apply to the face and neck.

skin polishing

All skin types look better after a weekly polishing treatment to slough off dead surface cells. In India, where a tropical climate means more oily skin and therefore a tendency to collect dust and grime, women have used home-made skin polishers for a long time.

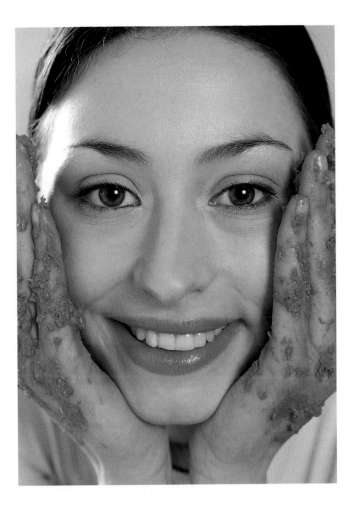

Every description of a mythological or legendary character in India has references to the skin. The lustre of the skin contributes to a divine appearance. Even in north Indian classical music each *raga* or modal melody is represented by a divine human form, with all the characteristics that listening to the *raga* are supposed to invoke. These ideas were first expressed in the *Natya Shastra*, a treatise

above
Women have always enjoyed the luxury of a rich and fragrant face-mask. Make your own at home using fresh ingredients such as sandalwood, orange juice and a very small pinch of turmeric.

on music and dance written around AD 300. Thus the *raga* 'Kaushika', a night melody, creates a mood of joyous abandon and is visualised as a woman 'with breasts like full moons, with skin like the lotus petal and bare thighs like banana trunks, who comes smiling and singing sweetly, perfumed with saffron'.

fenugreek facial scrub

According to Ayurveda, fenugreek seeds are a 'miracle spice'. They rejuvenate the body and contain steroidal saponins that resemble some of the body's own sex hormones.

2 tbsp fenugreek seeds

1 tbsp plain live yoghurt

Soak the fenugreek seeds in the yoghurt for an hour, then blend coarsely to a paste. Gently rub this on to the face and neck using circular movements and wash off after 15 minutes.

orange radiance facial scrub

This fragrant polisher will make your skin soft and radiant.

1 tsp dried orange peel (see *method*)

1 tsp oatmeal

3 tbsp rosewater

To make dried orange peel, finely grate fresh orange peel and allow it to dry naturally in an airy place till brittle: in wet weather it may be more practical to dry it in a very low oven. Mix it with the other ingredients, then gently rub on to the face and neck using gentle circular movements. Wash off after 15 minutes.

pineapple refining facial scrub

The enzymes in the pineapple soften and smooth the skin while the ground almonds slough off old skin.

1 tbsp chopped fresh pineapple

1 tsp ground almonds

Simply mix the ingredients together and rub on to the face and neck using gentle circular movements, paying special attention to areas prone to excess oil, such as the forehead, nose and chin. Wash off after 15 minutes

skin problems

My female ancestors have always believed that skin health is by and large hereditary. If your mother had a flawless complexion or was prone to acne, in all likelihood so will you. But heredity is not the whole story. Many skin problems are also caused by poor diet, bad circulation, not enough cleansing and a lifestyle which involves excessive smoking, excessive alcohol intake and even drug abuse. A lack of fresh air will also lead to blotchy skin.

acne Most beauticians agree that acne, which appears as a sheet of red pimples across the face, has much to do with the over-activity of the skin's sebaceous or oil glands and less with 'unhealthy' food we might eat (such as chocolates and crisps) or with dirt. Of course, a bad diet does aggravate the problem just as a good diet of fresh fruit and vegetables, eggs, meat, fish and milk promotes healthy skin from within.

Teenage acne is a condition that erupts due to an upsurge in hormonal activity during puberty. Unfortunately, there is very little that can be done, except to control it with diet or medicated lotions. Teenage acne usually quietens by the early twenties. Stress acne is more likely to spring up in the thirties and comes as large, single spots that are painful to touch and take a while to disappear. Women with a perfectly healthy complexion can find themselves with a problem skin overnight if they are stressed or over-worked. The occasional bout of painful acne around the time of menstruation is due to increased hormonal activity.

The first step towards keeping acne in check is to purify the blood. Ayurveda has many cures for this including the powerful-smelling but wonderfully rejuvenative garlic. One bulb a day soaked in vinegar (to lessen the smell) cleanses and renews the blood and regulates the digestion: eat the garlic and discard the vinegar.

Another, more pleasant blood purifier is water. Drink as much as you can throughout the day – beauticians recommend 2 litres (3½ pints) or 8 large glasses. It will flush out toxins through urine and help to keep the skin healthy. It must be pure water, though: drinks containing caffeine, such as tea, coffee and cola, actually have the opposite effect as they dehydrate the body.

My grandmother Sushila had a secret remedy for my acne-prone teenage cousins who could not bear to be seen by anyone and, on drives, would roll up the windows of their car for fear of being spotted by a friend. She would prepare a teaspoonful of onion juice, mix it with half a teaspoon of honey and advise my despairing cousins to apply this to the face twice a day, saying that the pungent element in onions would boost a sluggish circulation and heal the skin. She would also banish

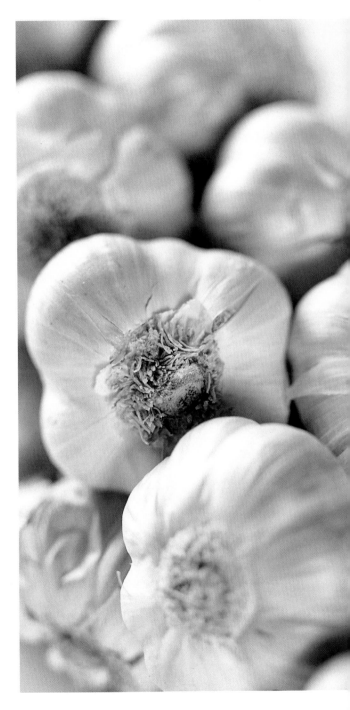

sugar and fried foods from their diet, murmuring rudely when they complained, that it would be impossible to find them husbands if their looks did not improve!

blackheads

Blackheads are not dots of dirt, but a mixture of secretions, the debris of old skin cells and bits of keratin, all coloured by melanin, the pigment which colours our skin and hair. This is why very fair people seem less prone to blackheads.

Thorough cleansing should stop some blackheads from forming, while steaming is the most effective way of getting rid of them. Steaming brings them to the surface of the skin from where they can be eased out with special extractors available at all chemists. Always close the pores with a mild astringent such as witch-hazel afterwards. My never-fail trick to keep blackheads at bay and tone my skin before a night out is to rub a wedge of juicy, red tomato over my face and neck for about five minutes and rinse it off. Tomato is very rich in vitamins A, B, C and E and contains amino acids and salts, such as citrates and tartrates, that give it a sour taste and make it a good astringent for the skin.

blemishes

Blemishes are usually temporary and can be caused by anything from strong sun and wind to an excess of alcohol. A light dab of either sandalwood or turmeric powder mixed in a little water should clear the problem. Both of these have unique antiseptic properties. Carrots, known for their high vitamin A content, are good for the eyes as well as the skin and make a wonderful treatment. Simply grate a carrot, squeeze out a teaspoonful of fresh, saffron-coloured juice and then wipe over the blemished areas. Rinse off after half an hour.

enlarged pores

Enlarged pores are caused mainly by the over-stretching of pores that then fill with excess oil. Any part of the body that stretches beyond its capacity may refuse to return perfectly to its original shape and size, and pores are no exception. The problem can be resolved temporarily by closing the pores with astringents, so that the skin looks toned. Buttermilk or watered-down yoghurt, a popular drink all over India known as *chaas* or *lassi*, works wonders, closing the pores to create the illusion of finely textured, perfect skin. Use it as a daily face wash and splash with cold water afterwards.

In many parts of northern India the summer is heralded by heaps and heaps of fresh, pale green cucumbers. Filled with juice, these are eaten with a light dusting of salt to make the intense heat bearable. Ice-cold cucumber juice used on the face and neck cools, refreshes and tones the skin and can be a real summer treat for the complexion.

moles

In India tiny, flat moles on the face and body are considered extremely sensual and desirable. Several poems written in the last twenty years describe the beauty of bow-shaped, luscious, ruby lips guarded by a mole placed discreetly beside them. In Indian folklore, stories tell of the perfection of the moon being somewhat balanced by the dark patches on it, and in the same way a mole by being an 'imperfection' in a beautifully perfect face, will deflect the 'evil eye' or the envious feelings of onlookers.

Leave moles alone unless they change shape or colour or begin to ache or bleed. If any of this happens, see a doctor.

make-up

Women have been using make-up for at least five thousand years. Their passion for and pursuit of beauty meant that they spent hours in front of a mirror, painting their faces and bodies. Today, the tradition is continued – although while body art and tattooing go in and out of vogue, make-up for the face is consistently popular,

Hindu temples built from around the sixth century AD and onwards, and particularly those at Konarak in Orissa, Khajuraho in Madhya Pradesh and at Halebid and Belur in Karnataka, are all decorated with stone sculptures of elegant women adoring themselves with jewellery and cosmetics. A finely chiselled stone pillar at the Halebid temple is embellished with an engaging dancer looking narcissistically into her mirror, her hair and robes nearly loosened as she applies kohl to her eyes.

The repertoire of classical Indian dance has countless songs dedicated to the long and lavish make-up routine followed by classical heroines. 'O lover! I wait for you with the kohl of the black night in my eyes, with the moonlike cool sandalwood painted on my breasts, the shimmer of rubies on my lips and a fire that can only blaze for you in my heart. But even the sandalwood burns my skin and the moon mocks me... for you do not come!' laments an anonymous, classical Sanskrit poem composed for dance.

Early make-up contained natural dyes from fruits, leaves and flowers. Henna coloured the lips and nails, kohl lined the eyes, while red lac from the lac insect and betel leaf juice were used to stain the lips and palms. Today, commercially produced cosmetics make up the Indian woman's toilette. As canvas does to a painting, so the skin provides the perfect backdrop on which to highlight the eyes and mouth. Good cleansing, toning and moisturising set the stage for the world of illusion that will follow.

foundation
Foundation or make-up base gives the impression of even-toned, blemish-free skin. Whether your skin is alabaster, chocolate or ebony, there is a right shade of foundation for you, and the fainter you apply it, the more natural it will look.

Foundation works best when applied with a damp sponge or with the fingers. Light, feathery strokes blend the colour into the skin (do not forget the neck) and fade it into the hairline and chest. Heavy foundation does not hide blemishes better. In fact it accentuates fine lines by accumulating in the creases and looks too theatrical and ageing in the glare of real life. A light veneer looks radiant and professional and helps to protect the skin from the harsh effects of weather. Change the foundation you use according to the season – light and warm in summer when the skin is more tanned and paler for fair winter skin.

To improve the shape of your face with make-up, look at it keenly in good light and decide what needs to recede and what needs emphasising. A broad nose, heavy jaws or double chin are all worth shading and shaping, whereas good, high cheekbones, the brow bone and the hollow above the upper lip should be highlighted. To slim a wide nose,

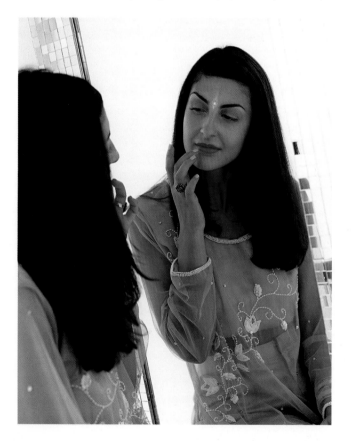

choose a foundation about two shades darker than your own and draw a line down either side of the bridge. Blend down towards your cheeks so the sides of the nose are darker than the bridge – ensure that no harsh lines remain.

blusher
The one item of make-up that will give an instantly healthy glow is blusher. Until a few centuries ago Indian women used a fine emulsion of *rakta chandan*, a red version of sandalwood with all its properties save the fragrance, to colour their cheeks. Blusher, as we know it today, can do a lot to shape the face. A sheer dusting is enough – too much will end up looking like a bruise. Experiment with your face to see how shading works for you. Applying blusher on the cheekbone can appear cherubic; just under it, chic. Select a colour that complements your complexion: pink if you are fair, coral or copper for tawny skin and wine for dark skin.

face powder
If you want your make-up to last, there are two things you can do. First splash ice-cold water on your face and neck after you have applied foundation to set the base. Gently pat dry and continue your routine. Second, seal your look with a fine dusting of loose face powder. Use a soft, fat brush and blow away any excess before you start on your face. Blend well to eliminate any powdery patches. Carry a compact of pressed powder with you – it is a great make-up reviver. Many women choose translucent over-tinted powder to give the face an evenly made up look without the burden of added colour.

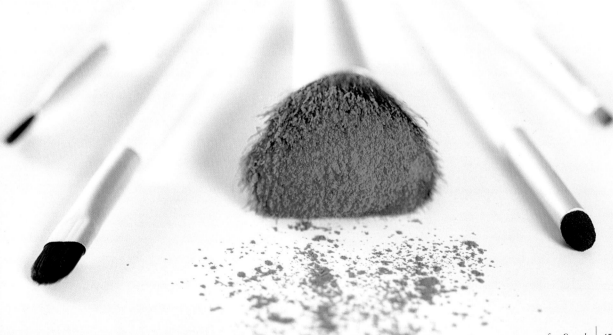

your skin and the weather

Changes in the weather can make our skin and hair behave in a dramatically different way. Soaring temperatures mean a shiny face and make-up that has to be rescued every few hours; a new frost heralds the arrival of extra moisturisers and creams on the dressing table. It is important to recognise the transformation of your skin from climate to climate. In India the seasons shift from extremely hot summers to very humid monsoons and lastly to the winter which is cold and bracing. Of course, India is vast and the weather in the north is completely opposite to that of the south. Being geographically closer to the equator and surrounded by the ocean on three sides, the triangular tip of south India is drenched in tropical heat and humidity. Here the skin tends to secrete more oil and perspiration that in turn cause

rashes and spots. Make-up seems to melt the minute you have applied it. In such weather choose powder based make-up that will last longer. South Indian women cool the skin with rosewater and sandalwood masks. It also helps to cleanse your skin thoroughly at least twice a day and dab on a little lemon juice diluted in water afterwards. If you can spray this on to your face and neck from a small spray pump, you will feel even more refreshed.

In places like New Delhi the weather swings to extremes. The dry, hot summer makes the skin feel parched and thirsty. Make-up forms blotches over dry patches and washing the face only aggravates the tightness of the skin. Hot breezes and the summer sun burn into the skin and eyes, so try to avoid going out in the strongest sunlight hours – between noon and tea-time. Moisturise frequently, with a product that contains an effective sunscreen. Use lip balm or coconut oil on the lips and choose cream-based make-up.

Srinagar in Kashmir nestles amid snowy peaks and pine-scented forests. Here the pure mountain air refines the skin and preserves its youthful glow. Snow has its own glare, which can be extremely harmful for the eyes and skin. Wear a good pair of sunglasses and never go out without applying sunscreen on your face and neck first.

winter skin

Dry skin needs extra nourishment in winter. A weekly oil massage (use almond oil) will revitalise the face and neck. Cleanse off with a ball of moist cotton-wool. Too much soap can cause havoc with dry skin, especially in winter, so cleanse with creams or oil instead. Chapped lips can be smoothed by keeping them covered in lipstick or gloss. Treat yourself to a creamy facial once a fortnight. Use fresh cream as a mask and rinse off after fifteen minutes.

summer skin

Keeping cool is the first thing on our minds in the summer. Go easy on the make-up and be sure to remove thoroughly whatever you do apply. Splash your face with cold water three to four times a day – but beware of too much soap, as it strips the skin of its natural oils. Wear only cotton clothes that are more absorbent and help perspiration to evaporate, and remember the golden rule of summer health: drink as much water as you can take.

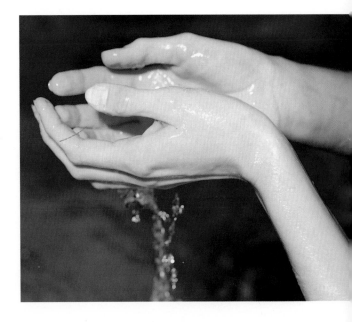

home facial

Sundays are for pampering and the best treat you can give your face is a home facial with creamy, fragrant confections that will leave it clean, glowing and ready for the week ahead.

1 Tie your hair away from your face, and wear something really comfortable. Cleanse your face with an oatmeal scrub (see page 36) and rinse off with warm water.

2 Now apply a thick moisturising cream (see page 38) to your face and neck. Wet your hands and work the cream all over your skin till it is smooth and silky. Use upward strokes from chin to temple, along laugh lines, over the nose from brows to temples. Make anti-clockwise circles on your cheeks with the pads of your fingers. Gently massage the cream into the skin around your eyes, including the lids, working from the inner corner of each eye, under it and then over the lid. Draw tiny circles on your forehead. Slap the jawline upwards. Smooth the skin of the neck upwards. Continue this massage for twenty minutes then pat dry with a soft towel. Do not wash the face yet.

3 This step is optional but will really refresh you. Steam your face over a pan of hot water (see pages 36–37) into which you can, if you wish, throw a handful of your favourite flowers. Ten minutes of steaming will open the pores so that they can be cleaned.

4 Now for the most delicious part. Whip up a really fragrant face mask (see pages 38–39) to suit your skin and slather it onto the face and neck. Cover your eyes with slices of cucumber and lie back for half an hour. Rinse off and pat on a toner. You will now glow with the lustre of a million suns!

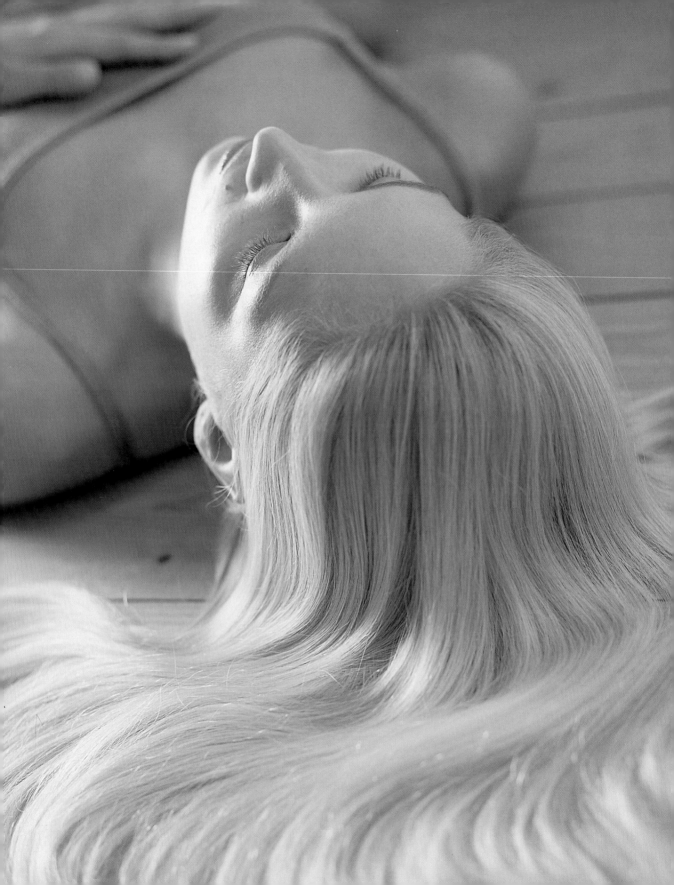

'Her long silken tresses like the lustrous plumage of a black swan, a simmering swarm of bees, spill down like the dark rain-swollen clouds...' *Shivalilamrit – hymn c.fourteenth century* AD, *describing the beauty of Parvati*

hair care

In Vedic times, thousands of years ago, women washed their hair with aloe vera gel, hibiscus flower juice and other fragrant herbs and then oiled it with coconut oil scented with jasmine, rose or sandalwood. They dried their hair over incense and the perfume would linger for days, scenting the air with even the slightest movement.

In those days styling the hair was also an essential part of a woman's daily beauty routine. There was the *kaparda* or shell-shaped hairdo, where a braid was twisted like a shell and worn on the right side of the head or two braids were looped on either side of the head; the *jata*, where the hair was braided and piled on the top of the head like a diadem; and the *dhammilla*, in which a long tube of hair was twisted and coiled around the head and the *stuka* or curls and *alaka* or locks were left loose to soften the face and enhance its charm.

Long hair has always been considered sensual and the classical romantic literature of India is peppered with heroines such as Sita in the *Ramayana* and Draupadi in the *Mahabharata* with endless, flowing tresses. Indian goddesses

are even named for their beautiful hair: Sukeshini, means 'the one with lovely locks' and Muktakesha 'she who has loose, dishevelled hair'. Ancient Hindu temples dating back several centuries depict celestial nymphs called *apsaras*, and dancers of the royal palace dressing their hair in many complex styles. These voluptuous figures wear jewelled ornaments on their forehead and along the parting of the hair. Strings of pearls are entwined around loose tendrils and thick, snake-like plaits dance jubilantly in the air as a twirling dancer is captured mid-movement in stone.

Many temple sculptures also show women shampooing their hair with an assortment of herbs and fruits. According to early Ayurvedic recipes, the herbs basil, *brahmi* (*centella*) and henna were beneficial to hair, and fruits like *amla* (*emblica*) gave it shine and softness. Even now herbs such as *bhringaraj* (*Eclipta alba*) which is known in Ayurveda as 'the king of the hair', and *brahmi* are used in hair products. *Bhringaraj* promotes hair growth, stops and reverses balding and premature greying and cools the head to keep the hair lustrous.

The hair has always had religious significance. Traditional Sikhs, whose religion forbids them from cutting their locks, still maintain a top knot bound by a turban. One of the first religious sacraments a Hindu child goes through is *chudakaran* or tonsure. Sushruta (c. AD 350), one of the fathers of Ayurveda, writes in his text Sarirasthana that 'shaving and cutting the hair and nails remove impurities and give delight and lightness, prosperity, courage and happiness'. The basis of the ritual of shaving a child's head, which usually takes place at the end of the first year of life, was for health and beauty.

The birth hair was removed and new hair grew back strong and thick. This ceremony, sometimes called *mundan* still prevails and is celebrated with much fanfare and feasting.

A head of shiny, well-maintained hair provides instant glamour to any woman. In India women have always considered long, thick hair beautiful and even today short hair is looked upon as a concession to a busy city lifestyle. In a tradition followed by their grandmothers and then their mothers, many working girls in the cities follow a special Sunday routine: they oil their hair well and plait it loosely, only to wash it the next morning. According to popular belief, this intensive nourishing treatment enhances the length and thickness of hair.

In the Hindu marriage rituals a mother-in-law presents her daughter-in-law with a *shringar* tray that contains all that she will need to decorate herself. This includes a silver comb, herbal hair oil and a jewelled ornament for the hair. In India, long hair is prized as an eternal symbol of feminine beauty. My own hair was long and cascaded like a sheet down my back all through my school days. My friends would touch it to feel the texture and strangers would ask me my beauty secrets. When I entered college, I felt the sudden need to appear cosmopolitan and had my hair cut according to the current 'hot' style. I will never forget the look of horror and disbelief on the faces of my family when I returned home that evening. They still have not completely forgiven me for betraying my wonderful locks and, much to my embarrassment, the incident is still recalled at family gatherings!

This powerful legend concerning Draupadi, the heroine of the Indian epic *Mahabharata* firmly establishes the value of the hair in an Indian woman's life. Draupadi, married to five brothers called the Pandavas, was lost in a game of dice

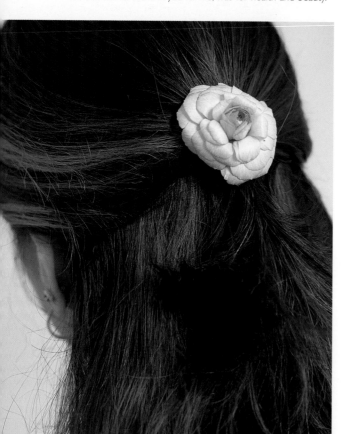

to the enemy-clan, the Kauravas. Duryodhan, the eldest of the Kauravas, who were cousins of the Pandavas, ordered Draupadi to be dragged to the court and disrobed in public. Dushasan, another Kaurava, gleefully set forth on his task, but Draupadi, a friend and devotee of Lord Krishna, appealed to him for help. Krishna, in all his divine glory, saved her honour by creating an endless sari that the wicked Dushasan could never ever take off. The fiery Draupadi could not bear this insult and announced in all her proud beauty, with yards and yards of fabric at her feet, that she would not tie her glorious hair again until she had anointed it with Dushasan's blood. Throughout the story she waits for the opportunity to avenge herself and writers have described her as walking through her palace with her loose hair swishing darkly around her knees.

The *Manu-Smriti* (c. AD 100–300), a doctrine written by Manu, the law-giver on Hindu jurisprudence, has a section laying down rules for women. One of these is that a married woman must not leave her hair loose in public, the reason being that her flowing tresses will lure new lovers who will seduce her away from her husband. For centuries afterwards, women were lead to believe that loose hair was a symbol of promiscuity. Today, of course, the *Manu-Smriti* is denounced by all modern Indian women as a symbol of misplaced patriarchy and preposterous domination.

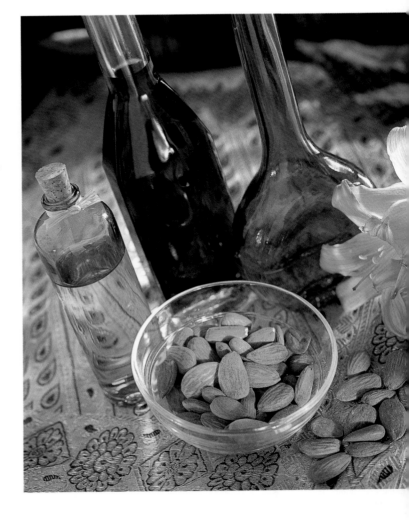

The contemporary Indian woman, however, still follows many home-tested hair routines. She regularly nourishes her hair with herbal oils, colours and conditions it with henna, shampoos it with extracts of fruits like *ritha* (also called soap nut because of the frothy, soapy infusion it gives when boiled in water), *amla* (*emblica*) and *shikakai* (known to promote healthy hair), and dries it over the smoke of a subtle incense stick to fragrance it. She leaves her hair loose, plaits it or ties it into a bun held together with ornaments. She buys fresh flowers from street vendors that she tucks into her plait, and fills her parting with red *sindoor* (used to draw the mark on the forehead) to announce that she is married. Today's Indian woman also cuts, perms, straightens, highlights or bleaches her hair to keep up with international fashion.

types of hair

Just as skin type varies from person to person, so too does the hair.

oily hair
The hair is kept healthy and lustrous by the natural oil produced by the sebaceous glands in the scalp. When these glands become over-active and produce excess sebum, the hair looks lank and lifeless and becomes greasy soon after washing.

Every woman goes through a 'greasy hair' time in her life during puberty, pregnancy or menopause. In India greasy hair is a persistent problem for many women because of the hot weather. The answer is to wash the hair every day with a mild shampoo. There is no truth in the myth that a daily wash will harm the hair. In fact greasy hair only attracts dust and grime, which make it and the scalp unhealthy. It is not a good idea, however, to be over-zealous in the shampooing of oily hair. This will just strip away essential as well as excess oils and leave the hair under-nourished.

Too much conditioner is also taboo – it flattens oily hair further. Nor should you activate your oil glands further by over-brushing the hair. Oily hair needs a low heat setting on the dryer to give it a finishing touch. Too much heat activates the sweat glands and makes even freshly washed hair sticky. Women with very greasy hair should oil their hair once a fortnight or so and leave it on for not more than half an hour. This will help to nourish the roots, which do not benefit nutritionally from the oil on the scalp.

A frothy hair pack once a week also helps to control the oil on your scalp. Beat the whites of two eggs till stiff and apply to the scalp and hair. Rinse off after half an hour. The protein in the egg will nourish while drying up the oil. Wash the hair thoroughly and use fresh lemon juice as a finishing rinse to eliminate the odour of raw egg and get the hair squeaky clean. Dilute a tablespoonful of juice in two cups of water and pour over the head after shampooing, then rinse away. A good alternative to lemon is ordinary vinegar from the kitchen cupboard. The acid removes traces of shampoo and smoothes down the cuticle of the hair, making it exceptionally shiny.

dry hair
Hair usually becomes dry because of a lack of oil and water content at the cellular level on the scalp. Dry hair looks dull and is prone to breaking and splitting because it is so brittle. This is why any brushing, combing and styling should be done very gently. The weather affects hair quickly and exposure to strong sun and wind will further dry it. Shampoo your hair only when necessary, using lukewarm water. Use a creamy conditioner to make dry, 'fly-away' hair manageable. Never brush hair when it is wet – it will break.

In India the oiling of the hair is a beauty routine followed by men and women alike and from the richest to the poorest of people. Every household has it own secret recipe for the

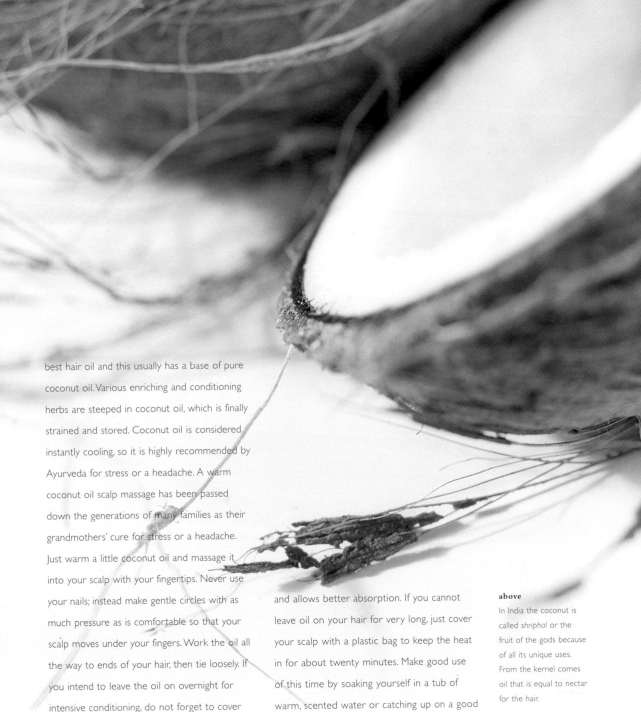

best hair oil and this usually has a base of pure coconut oil. Various enriching and conditioning herbs are steeped in coconut oil, which is finally strained and stored. Coconut oil is considered instantly cooling, so it is highly recommended by Ayurveda for stress or a headache. A warm coconut oil scalp massage has been passed down the generations of many families as their grandmothers' cure for stress or a headache. Just warm a little coconut oil and massage it into your scalp with your fingertips. Never use your nails; instead make gentle circles with as much pressure as is comfortable so that your scalp moves under your fingers. Work the oil all the way to ends of your hair, then tie loosely. If you intend to leave the oil on overnight for intensive conditioning, do not forget to cover your pillow with an old, thick towel.

Any kind of oil treatment benefits from the application of heat as this opens the pores and allows better absorption. If you cannot leave oil on your hair for very long, just cover your scalp with a plastic bag to keep the heat in for about twenty minutes. Make good use of this time by soaking yourself in a tub of warm, scented water or catching up on a good read. Olive oil is thicker than coconut oil but can also be used as a conditioning treatment for hair. It can also be left on for any length of

above

In India the coconut is called *shriphal* or the fruit of the gods because of all its unique uses. From the kernel comes oil that is equal to nectar for the hair.

time between twenty minutes and a couple of hours. My friend Smita suggests dry-massaging the scalp with the fingertips once a week. The movement encourages the sebaceous glands to secrete oil and improves circulation.

normal hair
Healthy, shiny hair has almost always had a good start because of well-balanced hormone levels and an ideal internal chemistry, but to keep it in fine condition you need to look after it carefully. Normal hair, however strong, can be damaged easily if not cared for properly. Wash gently only as often as needed and condition to keep it shiny. Conditioner has a positive electrical charge which makes the hair cuticles lie flat along the length. Only the hair needs conditioner – do not waste it on your scalp. All traces of conditioner must be rinsed away otherwise the residue will make the hair lank and sticky.

oil
Ancient Hindu texts on erotics, including the *Kamasutra*, devote entire chapters to the charms of courtesans and prostitutes. Along with the art most essential to her profession, as well as the affairs of the world, a courtesan was supposed to be knowledgeable and proficient in 'the sixty-four classical arts'. These included 'singing, flower arrangement, sorcery, gymnastics, training fighting cocks, carpentry, architecture, preparation of cosmetics for the face, oils for the hair…'

Oiling the hair has been a highly regarded ritual in India for at least five thousand years. Even today wise old women are convinced that regular oiling maintains the natural colour of the hair and prevents greying. Oil cools the head and promotes luxurious hair growth, whereas internal body heat does the opposite. Many of my own aunts still have jet-black hair even at the age of seventy!

Uma's nourishing hair oil
Here is my grandmother's recipe for a nourishing home-made hair oil. The tea stimulates the cells to produce new hair growth.

500ml (17fl oz) coconut oil

handful each of fresh or dried hibiscus, holy basil, marigold and balsam leaves

1 tsp tea leaves

Heat the oil in a deep *kadai* or wok till it is quite hot but not smoking. Take off the heat and drop in the herbs and tea leaves. Allow to steep for a day. Strain the oil into a pretty jar and use at least once a week.

oil for falling hair
The eucalyptus and clove oils in this preparation boost blood circulation that nourishes the root of the hair and prevents hair loss.

5 tbsp coconut oil

1 tsp eucalyptus oil

1 tsp clove oil

Mix the three oils together and gently rub into the scalp at night.

shampoos
Traditionally women in India have used herbs and fruits such as *ritha* (soap nut), *shikakai*, amla (*emblica*) and *neem* (*Azadiracta indica*) to wash their hair. *Ritha* nuts are so

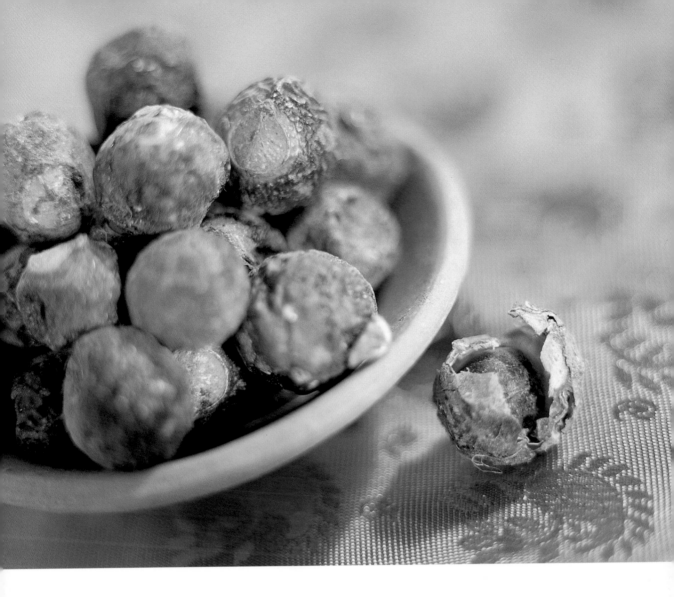

gentle, in fact, that they are also used to wash pure gold-embroidered, rich silk fabric.

ritha & lemon shampoo

The dried ritha nut makes an excellent but unlikely shampoo that can never harm your hair. You can substitute them with any part of the herb soapwort, which may be more easily available. Surprisingly both ritha, available at Indian shops, and soapwort clean the hair

thoroughly without producing lather. The lemon juice helps control oil secretion in a greasy scalp.

1 cup ritha nuts

1 tbsp fresh lemon juice

Soak the *ritha* nuts or soapwort in a cup of water overnight. The next day, strain the liquid and mix in the lemon juice. Apply to the hair in the usual way and rinse with water.

above

Village women in India swear by natural *ritha* nuts over the commercial shampoos used by their city sisters.

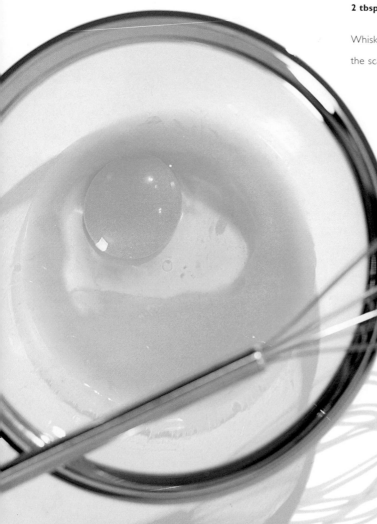

aloe vera shampoo

The herb aloe vera is known as *kumari* in Sanskrit, which means 'young virgin girl'. It is so named because it enhances femininity, of which one attribute is luxuriant hair. Aloe vera gel is available from natural health shops.

1 tsp pure aloe vera gel or

½ cup crushed aloe vera leaves

2 tbsp your regular shampoo

Mix the ingredients with a cupful of water and allow to stand for an hour. If using leaves, strain the mixture before use. Apply to the hair in the usual way and rinse with water.

orange shampoo (LEFT)

This shampoo is an excellent cure for excessive oiliness and the itchiness which results from it.

1 egg

2 tbsp fresh orange juice

Whisk together the egg and orange juice and massage into the scalp and hair. Leave on for fifteen minutes and rinse.

conditioners

Conditioners put the life back into dull hair and are simple to make at home. One of the most famous places of worship in south India is the Balaji temple at Tirupati. A great number of devotees, both men and women, come here from all over the country and ritually shave off their hair as a form of penance. Many people also believe, in a strange sort of way, that leaving behind a lock of one's hair at the temple will make the hair on the head healthy, luxurious and superbly conditioned. Some devotees even send a few hairs in a matchbox with whoever else is going on a pilgrimage to Tirupati. Fortunately, we will not have to go to that much trouble; here are some home-made recipes for conditioners.

henna conditioner for dark hair (RIGHT)

The addition of yoghurt and oil considerably reduces the ability of henna to colour. However, certain strong types of henna could overcome this, and in lighter hair the conditioner might leave behind some colour. The conditioner is therefore recommended only for dark hair.

1 cup henna powder

2 cups plain live yoghurt

1 tbsp olive oil

Stir all the ingredients together till the mixture resembles mud. Wearing gloves, work the henna into the hair, parting it and treating each section from the scalp down to the tip till the whole head is covered. Coil your hair on top of your hair if it is long or smooth it into wings from the side of your head to the back if it is short. Leave for an hour and wash off. You will need patience for this as washing dried henna out of the hair takes a little time.

my own super conditioner

When I was growing up in Mumbai, my parents owned a farmhouse in the verdant, waterfall-dotted slopes of the Sahyadri mountains. All kinds of wonderful herbs grew there and each weekend visit would find me bringing a basketful of freshly plucked herbs home to Mumbai to grind up into conditioning hair masks. I have never been able to achieve the same gloss and texture from any bottled conditioner.

handful each hibiscus, marigold, balsam, basil and

mint leaves

handful of rose petals

Grind all of these (or as many as you can find) in a blender with a little water till you get an emerald-green, coarse, sticky mixture. Apply this directly to the scalp and hair and leave on for at least an hour. Wash off thoroughly. Your hair is sure to gleam like gold!

hair problems

dandruff Most women go through a phase of dandruff at some stage in their life, when the skin on the scalp seems to come off in flakes. Sometimes this may happen as a result of too much exposure to wind and sun, a residue of shampoo being left behind on the head,

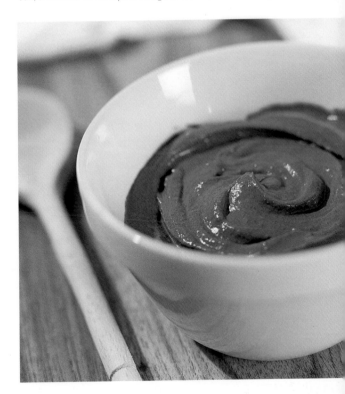

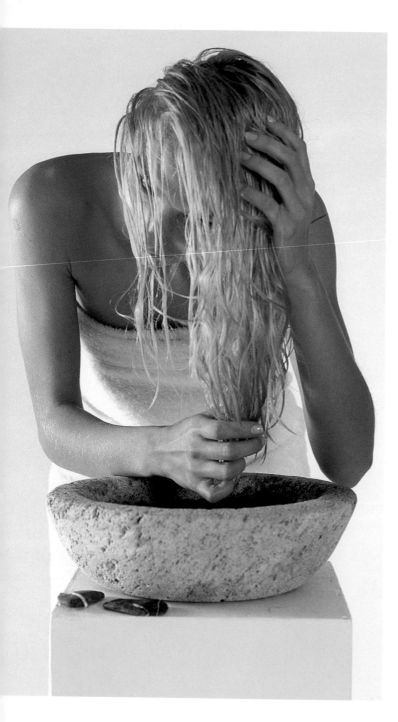

over-use of hair spray or the effects of a course of strong medicines. Like everywhere else on the body, the skin on the scalp also, needs to renew itself. When this skin cannot shed itself normally and accumulates on the scalp, we call it dandruff. When the scalp is dry, these flakes appear light and powdery, whereas on an oily head they seem to clog together. Keeping the hair and all your tools – brushes and combs – really clean is essential.

A quick way to control early dandruff is to rinse the hair after shampooing with a tablespoon of cider vinegar in a cup of water or with a strong infusion of parsley or raspberry leaves. Fresh apple juice massaged into the scalp also helps. The mild acid in apple exfoliates as well as checking excessive oil secretion. A nourishing hair pack that clears up dandruff can be made of four tablespoons rosemary infusion, an egg yolk and a pinch of borax: simply massage into the scalp before shampooing. Of course, occasional bouts of scurfiness can be cleared up with a relaxing massage with warm olive oil. Sometimes the scalp feels quite itchy without any actual flaking – in this case dabbing it with a ball of cotton wool soaked in witch-hazel will help.

far left

A quick rinse after shampooing is all it takes to maintain the gloss and colour of your hair. Vinegar, lemon juice or beer makes excellent rinses.

falling hair Losing seventy to eighty hairs each day is quite normal and regrowth is a continuous process. However, if you lose more than this and the amount of hair on your brush after regular brushing alarms you, it is time to sit up and take notice. Hair loss can be due to various factors – poor health, pregnancy, stress or certain medication.

Warm oil on the scalp nourishes it and helps prevent hair loss. Most importantly, a good protein diet that includes meat, fish, eggs, pulses (such as lentils) and dairy products strengthens the hair from the inside. Vitamin B is absolutely essential. The best source of this is brewer's yeast: one capsule a day should improve the condition dramatically. Iodine helps to boost the circulation to the scalp – eat plenty of iodine-rich seafood.

My grandmother's sure-shot recipe for falling hair was to apply to the scalp on alternate days for four days a tiny amount of castor oil and iodine. This is one of the most effective remedies that I know. It helps further to steam the head by wrapping it with a hot towel for half an hour. Shampoo the hair with an infusion of *ritha* or soapwort. Diluted lemon juice also works in stopping hair loss. I have also found that vitamin E helps my own hair to grow very fast. I have used oil with vitamin E or, as a dire measure, just broken a capsule of vitamin E on to my scalp and massaged it in. This never-fail trick has increased the length, thickness and shine of my hair within a month. With regular use (twice a week for six months) of this wonder vitamin, anyone can have lustrous hair like the Parvati whose 'plait is as thick, long and sinuous as a snake' (from the hymn *Shivalilamrit*).

premature greying The problem of premature greying seems to be accelerating as the world becomes more and more stressed and people seem to be on the go more and more of the time. Only about fifty years ago women in Europe would pour iron-rich red wine over their heads to stop hair colour from fading. Italian women would macerate the rind of a green orange in olive oil and massage the hair with this, whereas gypsy women in the west would happily drink a dose of nettle tea to keep their tresses jet black and shiny.

In India oiling the hair once or twice a week is considered the best prevention for greying hair, but once it is grey, the only answer is colouring. Oil infused with the herb *brahmi*, known for its power to darken, is used once a week from the age of five and women with youthful black hair at the age of seventy are not an uncommon sight. *Bhringaraja* (also called *maka*) oil is Ayurveda's answer for premature greying. It has been attributed with unique restorative properties that nourish and protect the hair. Both these oils are easily available at Indian shops.

split ends The only remedy for split ends is to snip them off. Excessive dryness leads to hair splitting and break-ing, with that typical bushy, frizzy and discoloured look. Keep the hair well nourished with a weekly deep-conditioning oil treatment and a nourishing hair pack of protein-rich egg yolk once every ten days.

hair colour 'Your skin has the lustre of silver, your hair is tinged with gold; whoever you fall in love with, my sweet, will become the richest man in the world,' sings a famous Urdu singer in a Mumbai concert hall as the audience dreams mistily of a utopia of love. Romantic Indian poetry has always described the allure of burnished skin and glossy dark hair.

Women all over the world wish to maintain the fresh colour of their hair for as long as possible. A temporary change of shade instantly 'lifts' the looks. The success of any colouring process will depend on the condition of your hair, whether it has already been coloured or chemically treated and whether it is oily or dry.

If your hair has a naturally beautiful colour, simple rinses will bring out gleaming highlights. Women in rural India often use a strong infusion of tea as a final rinse and I am told that in Jamaica, rum is added to the tea! An infusion of cloves in strong Indian tea can be used in the same way to darken greying hair.

Lemon juice is a natural bleach. Comb fresh lemon juice through damp hair and dry it in the sun. In a couple of weeks, depending on your hair's quality and its ability to catch colour, light brown hair will be streaked with clear, gold highlights.

Saffron, the most exotic of spices, is a natural colourant in Indian food and an infusion used as an after-shampoo rinse will most certainly give red tones to the hair. Steep a handful of dried marigold flowers in the infusion to intensify the effect.

The most popular hair colourant in India is henna, which comes from the lacy bush of the same name. This grows all over India and plucking and drying the leaves is a cottage industry run almost entirely by women. The olive-green, dried leaves are powdered and packed for sale. In fact, it is so easily available, economical and effective, that some men use it to colour their greying or white beards flaming red, as an adver-tisement for their devotion to personal grooming.

Several types of henna are available: some stain black, others give a cherry or walnut hue. The most natural one (with no additives like other herbs) should give a colour somewhere between red, orange and copper depending on your hair's colour and condition. Use on fair or white hair will result in a bright, carrot colour. Henna colours skin and hair immediately, the colour growing deeper as the henna dries.

To make a henna pack for the hair, mix henna powder with hot water so that it resembles thick, gooey mud. Henna is a permanent dye, so use gloves to stop your fingers and nails from staining. Part the dry hair with a plastic comb and apply the paste to the roots (taking care not to stain the skin around the hairline), working down to the ends of the hair. Continue until you have finished the entire head. Coil the hair away from the face and allow to dry before rinsing – you might need several applications to achieve the desired effect. Henna fades as it grows out, so there is no problem of roots showing. It also has a strong but delightfully herbal fragrance that lingers in the hair for a few days. Mixing the henna with tea or coffee, instead of water, makes the colour more intense.

extra-rich henna pack

This pack gives fiery, polished-wood tones to light to medium brown hair and ripe plum glints to dark brown or black hair.

About 1 cup henna powder (the quantity will depend on the length of your hair)
cold strong coffee or tea as needed to mix
1 egg

Mix together all the ingredients to form a thick paste, taking care to use cold tea and coffee, otherwise the egg will be scrambled! Leave on the hair for an hour and wash off.

far left
Various types of henna powders, depending on the different species of plant or the added ingredients in them, are available in the market. Egyptian and Indian henna are particularly popular.

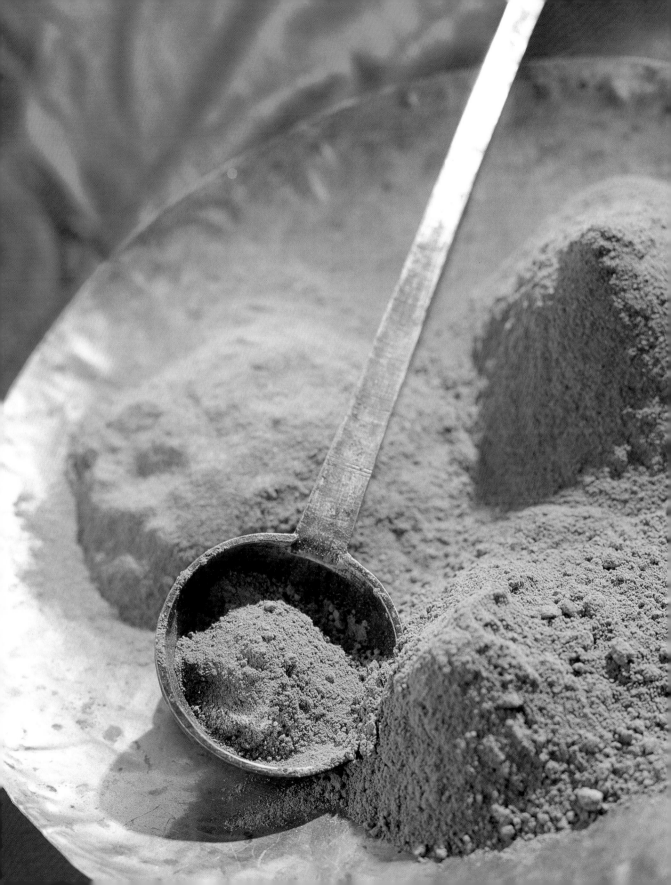

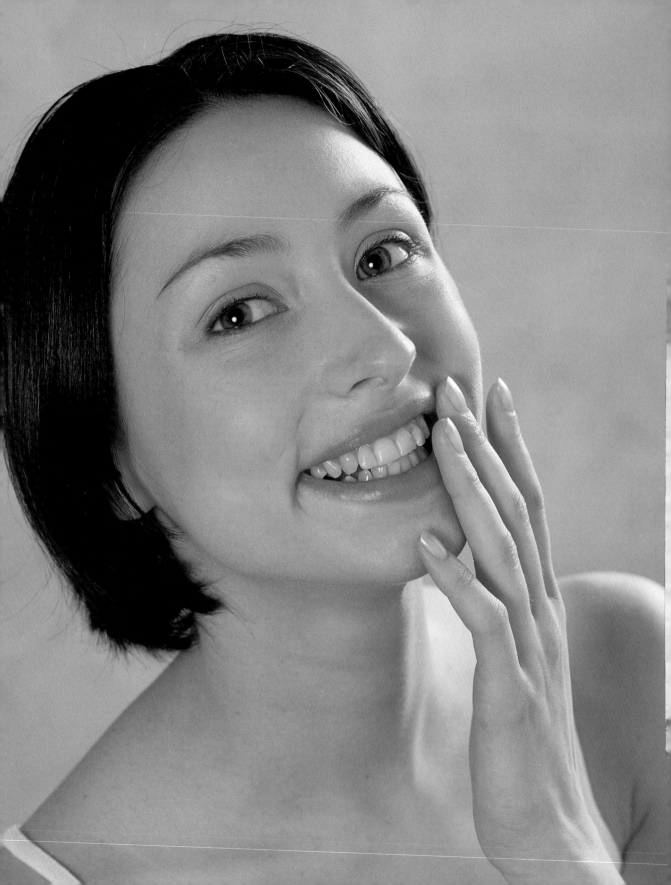

'The mother of the world smiles revealing her perfect teeth like a row of white swans, When she speaks, jewelled stones rain from her mouth, Her lips are like a bow, they are red and tender like full seeds of a pomegranate…' *Shivalilamrit*

mouth & teeth

Hindu mythology is based on the great trinity of gods named Brahma the Creator, Vishnu the Preserver and Shiva the Destroyer. Each has a consort who is the embodiment of energy and power. Brahma's wife is Saraswati, who is the goddess of speech and music and the inventor of the Sanskrit language. She is depicted as a fair young woman in white silk clothes holding a lute and a book and accompanied by a swan. She is still worshipped by singers and orators before they walk on stage. She rules over the spoken word and therefore is empress of the mouth and the speech faculties.

A popular Indian bedtime story is that of baby Krishna and his mother Yashodha. One day Krishna was playing near the river when he picked up a handful of earth and put it, as babies often do, in his mouth. His mother rushed up ready to admonish him and prise it out, but when he opened his mouth, she was speechless with shock. For inside was the entire universe: the planets, the stars, the moon and the sun, all spinning to a secret cosmic rhythm. His mother realised that this was no ordinary boy. He was divinity himself.

Ancient Hindu texts called the *Vedas* liken the mouth to a universe because of the limitless thoughts that are spoken through it. The mouth is one of the most expressive parts of the body. In ancient Hindu literature, heroines have been attributed with luscious mouths that are compared to lotuses, rose petals, rubies and pomegranates. According to the *Kamasutra*, a good lover is required to have teeth that are equal, pleasingly bright, capable of being coloured (with betel leaf or *paan*, which stains the mouth red and is traditionally considered to be extremely sensual), of proper proportions, unbroken and with sharp ends'. The defects of the teeth are described as being 'blunt, protruding from the gums, rough, soft, large and loosely set'.

The shape of the mouth too is considered to reveal your personality. Thin lips generally denote a mean, selfish temperament whereas full lips and a wide mouth signify generosity and sensuality. Kissing, for which the mouth must be fragrant and inviting, is also dealt with in great detail in the *Kamasutra*, which states: Kissing is of four kinds, viz. moderate, contracted, pressed and soft, according to the different parts of the body that are kissed…' Although India's ancient Hindu temples are full of couples kissing passionately, society in general is extremely modest about the public display of affection.

This reserve is nowhere in evidence at the end of a Hindu wedding when the bride and groom are invited to play certain cheeky games much to the delight of the onlookers. One of these involves a clove held by the girl between the teeth; the groom has to pry it away from her delicately with his own teeth. The ribaldry and innuendoes aimed at the newlyweds can only be imagined, especially as most marriages in India are still 'arranged' and so this would be the first time the couple have touched each other.

It is also the first time that the couple share each other's *jootha* or are 'sullied with saliva'. Indians have a very strong aversion to 'touch with their mouth what others have touched with their mouth'. Orthodox Hindus still do not drink by putting a glass to their lips, instead they hold it high over their upturned mouth and pour the fluid in. They do not share pieces of food or eat off the same plate. This rule is only relaxed for one's spouse and children.

Very traditional Hindus also have highly elaborate customs for cleansing the mouth. A twig from the *neem* tree, known for its medicinal properties, is used to clean the teeth in the morning. The fingers are used with a pinch of salt or finely roasted tobacco to massage the gums and teeth. A tongue scraper, which is a slim, curved, metallic bow, is used to refresh the tongue and remove all 'fur' from its surface. The mouth is then rinsed with fresh water several times. All Indians take particular care to rinse their mouth after each meal. This keeps the teeth healthy and the breath fresh.

a fragrant mouth

All of us at some time or other are concerned whether our mouths smell clean and fragrant. Bad breath is off-putting and can cause a great deal of embarrassment. In India, Ayurveda and personal hygiene habits have both had to respond to the highly spicy cuisine that can give rise to foul breath. Onions, ginger and garlic all leave an unpleasant odour that worsens with the passage of time.

Bad breath can also be an important symptom of something more serious. Tooth decay and gum infection can creep in so slowly that you may not even be aware that you have bad breath. One of the major culprits is plaque, a sticky, transparent film of harmful bacteria that is constantly being formed in the mouth. The bacteria themselves are not dangerous, but if allowed to remain, they organise themselves into colonies, producing toxic enzymes that eat into gum tissue and cause disease. Telling signs are puffy, sore gums, which bleed on brushing. Plaque also builds up layer by layer to form tartar. All this results in foul breath and the teeth can eventually becoming loose and fall out.

The key to a good mouth is cleanliness. Brush twice a day and rinse the mouth frequently, after anything you eat. Adults have thirty-two teeth each with five sides that need cleaning. Dentists recommend using a soft or medium toothbrush and a non-abrasive toothpaste, and, however careful you might be, a six monthly visit to a dentist for professional cleaning should be a priority.

We all know that sugar is bad – it combines with certain strains of plaque bacteria and forms dextran, a sticky substance that helps bind plaque to the teeth. A traditional Indian meal does not end with a dessert; sweets are eaten along with all the other courses. Instead, the meal is rounded off with *chass*, a thin drink made with a tiny amount of yoghurt stirred into water to which a few grains of salt may be added. This helps to wash the teeth and dislodge food particles from between them.

A mouth freshener is mandatory after an Indian meal. The most traditional one eaten all over India is *paan*, a betel leaf stuffed with cardamom, cloves, coconut and betel nut and folded into a neat triangle. *Paan* shops are found on every street corner and their owners take great pride in decorating them and keeping each tiny metal pot of ingredients gleaming. Each shop-owner has his own secret recipes that have been handed down through the generations. At a north Indian wedding feast the bridal couple is served a *palangtod paan*, literally a 'bed-breaking *paan*', that is filled with all sorts of secret aphrodisiacs.

The Gujaratis in western India have a custom of serving several kinds of *mukhwas* in a silver box with individual compartments and tiny spoons. *Mukhwas* literally means 'mouth fragrances' and is made of a mixture of roasted fennel seeds or aniseed, menthol, coconut, chips of betel nut, poppy seeds, melon seeds and cardamom powder. The recipe for *mukhwas* varies from house to house. *Supari*, another Indian mouth freshener, consists of little flakes of betel nut, the hard, dried fruit of betel palm, soaked in menthol and dried again. They are sometimes coated in *varq* or pure silver leaf to make them look attractive.

below
Indian mythology often likens the ruby red lips of goddesses and heroines to the seeds of the pomegranate, a fruit considered to be a symbol of prosperity.

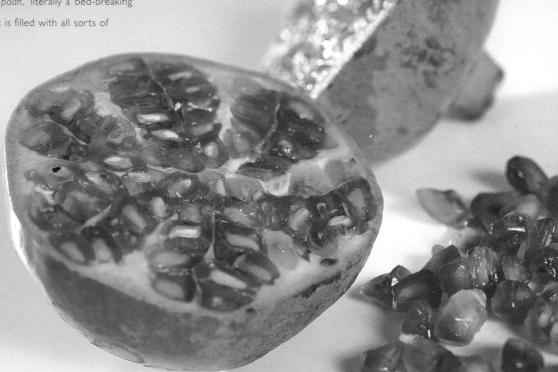

The Mughal queens who reigned over north India beside their husbands from AD 1200 to 1700 had more luxurious mouth fragrancers. As they reclined on flat bolsters on creamy marbled terraces, their robes rippling in the cool northern breezes, handmaidens would serve up tiny gold cups of rosewater from time to time, along with a spittoon. The royal ladies would discreetly rinse their mouths with the rosewater and the sullied spittoon would quietly be replaced by a fresh one.

Rosewater is still used as a mild mouthwash. Dilute four tablespoons in a cup of water and rinse the mouth, gargling thoroughly to wash the teeth and gums well. A mixture of 5 drops of peppermint spirit (available from chemists) in a cup of water is also quite effective. Clove oil (grandmother's remedy for a toothache), similarly diluted, also takes care of foul breath. A quick way to eliminate transitory odours caused by strong-smelling foods is to chew on any of the following: cardamom, cloves (be careful of the hot, sharp taste), aniseed, fennel seeds, mint leaves, holy basil leaves, an apple, carrot or cucumber. All of these also aid digestion, which affects the breath directly. Every mother tells her children that a good digestion means a healthy body signified by clean breath. Yoghurt is one of the best digestives you can have. The bacteria and enzymes in live (bio) yoghurt keep the internal system in tip-top condition.

Morning breath can be refreshed with a cardamom coffee, an old-fashioned remedy used in the misty Nilgiri hills in south India, where coffee plantations and a cultured colonial lifestyle happily co-exist. Grind a few coffee beans

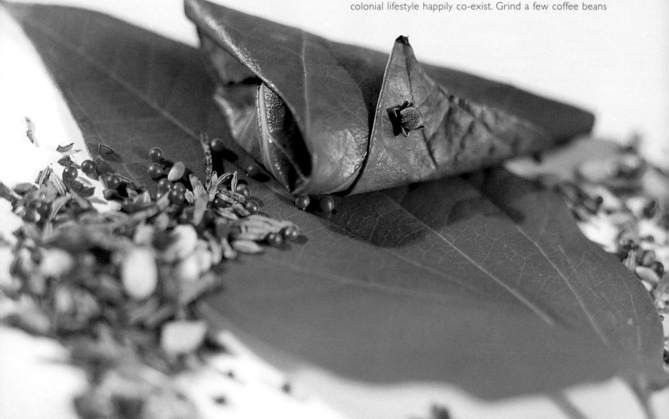

with seeds from a pod of cardamom and brew them into an invigorating cup of coffee to be drunk without milk as soon as you wake up.

the lips

One of the most alluring features of a woman is her lips – the shape, the texture, the pout can all draw attention in an instant. Add a soft smile to this picture and it becomes even more attractive. My grandmother Uma was an institution in herself, always surrounded by people who sought her advice and company as well as sharing their love and care with her. I'm sure that it was her happy, relaxed and ready smile for everyone that made them want to be near her. Even the most beautiful woman looks decidedly unappealing if her mouth is tight with anxiety, jealousy or hate. A smile lifts the face and will make people wonder what you are smiling about, adding to your mystery. Not only that, it also signifies that you are enjoying life and are supremely confident.

Lips respond to the weather and elements extremely quickly. An Indian summer or a frosty winter, harsh winds or strong sunshine can all make the lips dry and chapped. Lips need to be well lubricated at all times – simple Vaseline will usually do. This is especially true if you are outdoors a lot, sunbathing,

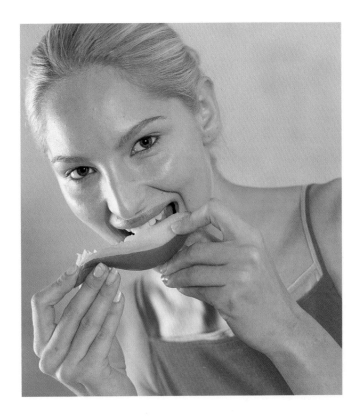

swimming or even just walking around. Women who work in the rice fields of south India, where the sun is at its fiercest, protect their lips with a fine gloss of coconut oil which is extremely gentle and nourishing. You can substitute this with olive oil, which may be more easily available in the West. To protect your lips in very cold weather try a combination of honey and rosewater, but do not be tempted to lick it off! I found the following recipes in an age-old cook book that gives handy hints for the judicious Indian housewife of the early 1900s.

left

Paan or a betel leaf stuffed with fragrant fennel seeds, coconut shavings, sugar balls, cardamom seeds and rose petal jam is eaten after an Indian meal as a mouth freshener.

coconut oil lip balm

2 tbsp grated beeswax

2 tbsp coconut oil

1 tsp almond oil

Melt the beeswax and coconut oil in a heatproof bowl
placed over a pan of hot water and whisk in the almond oil.
Remove from the heat, pour into a glass jar and allow to set.

rose lip protection cream (BELOW)

2 tbsp grated beeswax

2 tbsp almond oil

1 tsp rosewater

1 tsp honey

Melt the beeswax as above, then beat in the oil. Remove
from the heat and stir in the rosewater and honey till well
blended. Pour into a jar and allow to set.

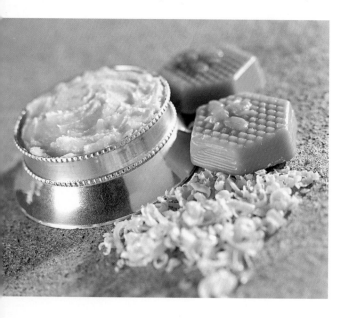

make-up

What woman is not attracted by rich, shiny lipstick? It
colours, highlights and corrects the form of the lips and is a
beauty aid that is available in plenty everywhere. Learning
to shape your lips with make-up is difficult and requires
practice – subtlety is the key, because a too-perfect,
conspicuous mouth will only look contrived.

Thin lips can be made to look larger, but not merely by
extending the lipstick beyond the edges of the lips. A
natural way to do this is to put a light smear of foundation
all over the lips and then draw an outline just outside the
natural lip line. The peaks on the top lip as well as the
curves of both lips can be emphasised a little, but leave the
corners of lips alone. Use a lighter shade of lipstick in the
centre of the lips and add lots of shine with a gloss. This
'opens' the lips and draws attention to them.

To tone down full lips cover them with a light veneer of
foundation, then draw an outline just inside the natural lip
line, stopping short at the corners. Fill in the colour in the
middle, using the same shade as the outline, but leave the
corners natural. Steer clear of lip gloss. Gloss can be used
to 'draw out' a reticent lower lip – but do not use it on
the upper lip at all.

Some women have lips that droop at the corners,
giving them a melancholy expression. Change this by
extending the outline of the lower lip at the corners.

An amazing variety of lip colours is available today, but
the more natural shades of pink, coral and russet still
look superb anywhere. Even in ancient India the
preferred colour was red from *lac* dye and all passing
fashions for blue, green, purple or black lipsticks are
usually only that.

the teeth

Before toothbrushes or toothpastes, people all over the world used the bark or twigs of certain medicinal plants to keep their teeth clean. One end of the stick was chewed till it became soft and frayed and this was carefully inserted between the teeth to remove all plaque. Each country had its own preferred plant: in the British Isles it was elderwood twigs, whereas in India it was *neem* sticks. According to Ayurveda, *neem* is a superlative cleanser and detoxifier. It heals sores and mildly disinfects the gums. *Neem* is used in several Indian commercial toothpastes.

Until a few hundred years ago, toothache was a common problem – dentists were unheard of and methods of extracting rotting teeth were primitive. Of course whitening and disinfectant powders were made at home from ingredients such as salt, charcoal, soot or burnt tobacco, and these are still used by some people in India, who would vote for them over any modern toothpaste. A sensible preventive measure is the application of eucalyptus oil on the gums. For toothache, a small ball of cotton wool soaked in clove oil and pressed into the cavity of the offending tooth can be used. Indian mothers mix clove oil and honey to apply locally on a baby's gums during teething.

The following toothpowder and whiteners can be used in performing a weekly spring-cleaning of the teeth, in addition to your twice-daily brushing regimen.

cinnamon toothpowder

This is especially good for sensitive teeth that tingle, as it helps make them strong.

2 tbsp cinnamon powder

4 tbsp arrowroot

pinch of pepper

Mix the ingredients to a paste with water. An even more powerful effect will be achieved if you use mint juice instead of water and add a pinch of salt once in a while for really deep cleaning. The salt acts as an abrasive and whitens the teeth. To make mint juice, blend ½ cup fresh mint leaves with 1 tablespoon water in an electric blender, or pound in a mortar, then strain.

lemon tooth whitener

Lemon is a natural bleaching agent and bicarbonate of soda a very gentle abrasive.

1 tsp bicarbonate of soda

½ tsp salt

lemon juice to mix

below

The East India Company began the cultivation of cloves in India around 1800, but even before then, they found their way into the country and were used among other things as a sure cure for toothache.

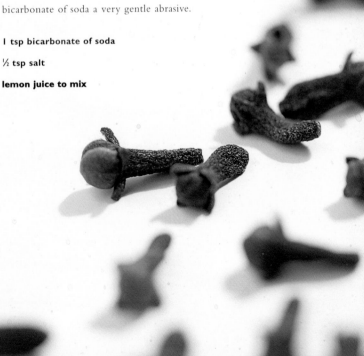

Blend all the ingredients and massage into the teeth and gums with your finger. Alternatively, put a little of this paste on your toothbrush and brush normally.

warning Although, white, pearly teeth are sought after, it is not a good idea to make frequent use of abrasive agents or commercial whiteners that will strip away enamel along with the tartar and plaque.

brushing

The importance of correct brushing cannot be over-emphasised. Your toothbrush must be soft enough, but not too soft, to work around the curves of the teeth and enter the crevices and irregularities. The bristles should be dense and preferably made of nylon for the required stiffness. You can now also buy toothbrushes with tufts of varying lengths that are claimed to be more more efficient at reaching awkward places. Replace your toothbrush as soon as the bristles start to splay and bend backwards upon themselves. If you are brushing properly without applying too much pressure, your toothbrush should last you two to three months.

When using commercial toothpaste, choose a fluoride one, so that over time some of the mineral will be absorbed, protecting the teeth against decay. (Do check with your dentist whether your local water is already fluorinated. If it is, they can advise you about your choice of toothpaste.) Remember to brush every surface of your teeth. Start on the lower jaw from the back. Learn to make tiny circular motions covering the sides and the top of each tooth. Work to the front, then go over to the other side. Do this to the upper teeth as well. For the front, close the teeth and brush up and down as opposed to in a horizontal movement. Hard brushing does not mean clean teeth – you may start up a problem of bleeding gums and still leave a lot of plaque behind. Softly brush your tongue to remove morning 'fur' and any bacteria that cause bad breath. Now rinse the mouth well with water.

Dental floss will get to places that a toothbrush cannot reach and flossing should be done once every two or three days. Remember that overzealous cleaning of the teeth will only weaken them. Also, however great the temptation, never dislodge food particles with a pin or sharp object – you might pierce the gum and thereby create a convenient environment for bacteria to breed and cause infection.

ulcers & sores

According to Ayurveda, most mouth ulcers are a result of eating the wrong types of food which have an excess of one element and a deficiency of another. Small white or red spots in the mouth or in corners of the lips, which burn and ache on touching, come up suddenly and take a while to disappear.

All Indians are brought up to know which health problems can be caused by eating foods that have 'hot' or 'cold' properties. Mouth ulcers are considered to be directly caused by 'hot' foods such as meat, alcohol, pineapples and garlic that create internal heat in the body, leading also to skin eruptions. Our family recipe for mouth ulcers was very efficient and tasted delicious.

remedy for mouth ulcers (RIGHT)

1 cup cold milk

2 tbsp rosewater

½ tsp pure sandalwood powder

Mix together all the ingredients and drink at bedtime for at least a week.

My mother would supplement the above cure by rubbing tiny amounts of calendula ointment, known for its healing properties, on the sore. Honey too has great curing properties and works as a disinfectant.

Many doctors today believe that a deficiency of vitamin B causes mouth ulcers. I think grandmother was already in the know – no wonder we were given extra doses of peas, potatoes and cereals. Liver is also a very good source of the vitamin.

Another useful piece of advice was 'Drink plenty of water and cool down the body.' I remember glasses of water, sometimes flavoured with cooling sandalwood, rose or *khus* (vetiver), being served up hourly, while dinner was yoghurt and rice without any spice or salt. I still cannot look at yoghurt and rice without thinking fondly of my grandmother. She swore by it as a cure for every conceivable internal ailment, claiming that it was *thump*, a local dialect word that can be roughly translated as 'peaceful'.

Mouth ulcers tend to occur when we are under undue stress and blood circulation becomes sluggish. Try to combat this, and prevent that 'run-down' feeling, by practising deep breathing, exercising regularly and making time for relaxation.

below

As a young girl I did not mind suffering the discomfort of a mouth ulcer because it meant that I could drink this delicious milky remedy, flavoured with rosewater and sandalwood.

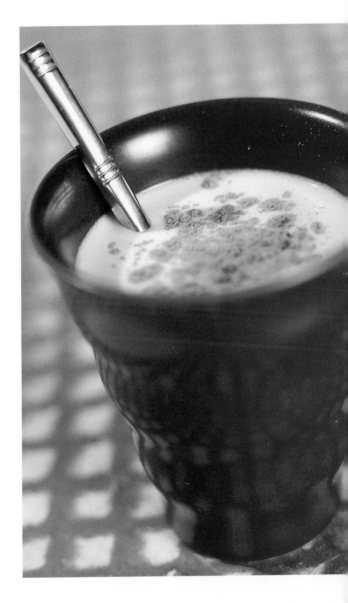

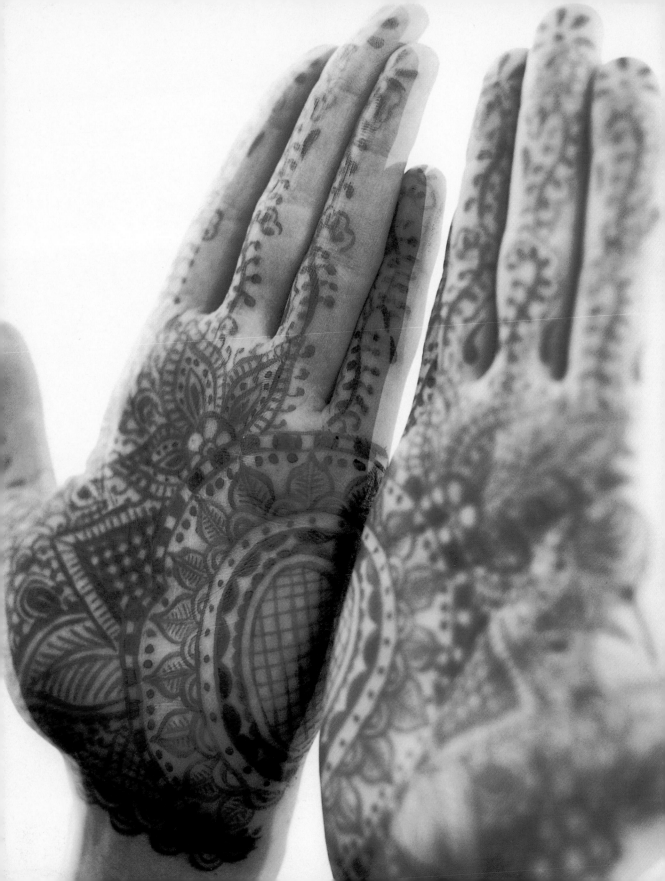

'Her hands, like white lilies, are givers, Givers of wealth, peace, joy...'

hymn to goddess Lakshmi

hands & feet

Both hands and feet have had special significance throughout Indian history. In Sanskrit the hand is called *hasta* which means 'that through which we experience'. In India the hands speak a language of their own and most Indians make expressive gestures as they converse. Drivers make wild signs to each other that are no part of the Highway Code and in the Indian classical dance, the *mudras* or hand movements express entire stories from the vast ocean of Indian mythology. The fingers curl into a lotus shape, straighten out to form a flag, undulate to copy the ocean waves and quiver like a flash of lightning. The story unfolds as the feet stamp out the rhythm in the music, the hands make alluring shapes and the eyes speak the emotion. The Hindu marriage is considered complete when the parents of the bride 'give her away' to the groom. The bride's father places her hand in the groom's palm while her mother pours a little water from the River Ganges, which is considered sacred, and places a holy basil leaf on the joined palms to signify that she is now truly his.

The Sanskrit word for foot is *pada*, which means 'the point of contact with the earth' and 'that which is a source of nourishment to the physical body'. Five thousand years ago the inhabitants of India believed that the feet drew

energy from the earth almost like the roots of a tree and hence the custom of walking around barefoot came into existence. A footprint was considered to have all the qualities of the owner. Thus a king could be vanquished in war if the dust from his footprints was scattered in the wind, a thorn pierced into the footprint of a runaway could make him stop, and rituals performed over the footprint of a maiden could win her love.

To this day the footprints of great people are revered. Images of footprints of gods and saints are crafted out of silver and enshrined with great pomp and ceremony. Buddhists worship the footprint of Buddha and the festival of Diwali sees many tiny footprints painted outside each Hindu house – these symbolise the arrival of the goddess Lakshmi, the harbinger of good fortune. According to mythology, the death of Lord Krishna was due to the folly of a hunter named Jaras who mistook the god's foot for a nimble deer and shot a poisoned arrow through it.

Orthodox Hindus never wear their footwear into the house as they consider it a temple, and taking shoes inside would be equal to defiling it. In fact in every traditional household, the lady of the house will ceremonially wash the feet of her guests outside the home. This ritual is repeated at Hindu weddings when the parents of the bride wash the feet of the bridegroom with scented water. The feet of the temple deities too are washed daily, to honour the gods and to seek their blessings.

The feet and footsteps are firmly ingrained into several Hindu rituals, including that of marriage. A marriage is said

henna paste, almost like small icing bags. At a modest henna party they can do up to forty pairs of hands! The bride of course takes longer as her designs are the most intricate.

In some parts of India, especially around West Bengal, the hands and feet of goddesses and brides are painted with a bright red dye called *alta*. All Indian classical dancers are

'She walks gracefully like a swan, her anklets ring out the music of the universe and wherever her beautiful feet step, red lotuses grow…' *Shivalilamrit*

to be complete, irrevocable and legal only after the *sapta-padi* or seven steps. The groom leads the bride by the hand as she places her foot on seven little heaps of uncooked rice. Each step represents a blessing, namely food, strength, wealth, happiness, progeny, cattle and devotion. The groom promises to look after his bride and asks her to be his friend and partner in looking after among other things, his family and the environment. When the new bride enters her husband's home, she first stops at the front door, prays for marital bliss and overturns a little silver cup of rice into the house with her right toe, signifying that she has brought prosperity and good fortune with her.

In all these ceremonies the decoration of the hands and feet takes on special meaning. Women of all faiths – Hindu, Sikh and Muslim – love embellishing their hands and feet with henna. A day before the celebration, women of the house, friends and neighbours come together to celebrate and have their hands and feet painted with flowers, curls, flourishes and creepers. A professional henna artist is invited with her assistants. They bring with them tiny cones of

painted in the same way, to draw the attention of the audience to the intricate hand gestures and foot-stamping rhythms. *Alta* washes off easily and is often used in place of the more permanent henna.

Jewellery has always been an Indian woman's passion. Even today her hands and feet are richly decorated with ornaments. In some orthodox sects among Hindus and Muslims, the only two men allowed access to the women of the house are the tailor and the bangle seller. Only the latter can touch women's hands while measuring them for the right size of bangle and can slip the bangles on to their wrists without any fear of the family sword being driven through his heart by the menfolk! Various bangles are worn on the wrist, each with its own name and etched with symbols like flowers, elephants, conches, lions, creepers and wheat. All these symbolise prosperity, divinity and fearlessness. Gold and silver bangles interspersed with glass ones, are a symbol of marriage.

Rings are symbols of love and are studded with precious and semi-precious stones from all over India. Turquoise, amethyst, topaz, peridot and garnet all vie with each in jelly-like sparkling confections.

Shiny anklets and toe-rings put shimmer on the feet. Indian dancers wear heavy bells on their feet just as Lord Nataraja, the god of dance, did when he performed the mythical cosmic dance. Each bell has a tiny bead within and twenty-seven such bells are woven on to a velvet belt tied to the foot with long strings. According to the *Natya Shastra*, the ancient treatise on dance written by Bharata between AD 100 and 300, the twenty-seven bells represent the same number of *nakshatra* or celestial stars that govern the lives and circumstances of everyone on earth, and the velvet used must be blue to represent the heavens. During the dance the dancer is a symbol of Nataraja and is attributed with his divine energy.

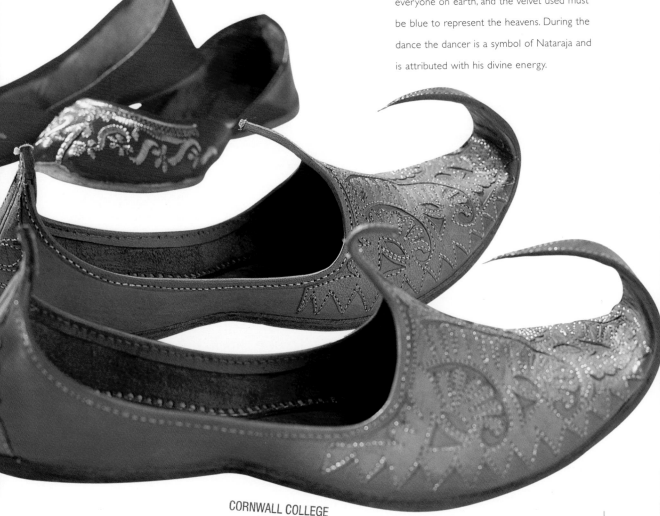

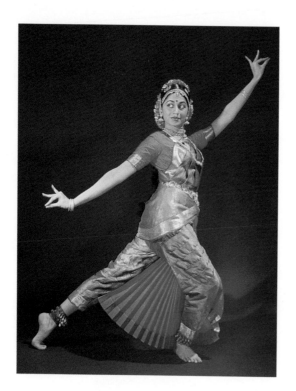

All Indians are great believers in fortune and destiny and every village has its own palmist. Sometimes his working partner is a little green parrot who selects fortune cards for a gullible customer. However, the science of palmistry is as old as the *Vedas* and experienced palmists can decipher the lines on the palm to reveal exact dates and circumstances about one's life.

Thousands of years ago the people of India believed that the hands were conductors of divine energy – giving strength and healing, but capable of wounding or killing too. The handprint also imbibes the powers of its owner and, to this day, people in rural areas dip their hands in dye and stamp their prints at the front door to protect the house from evil.

care of the hands

The hands usually show signs of ageing faster than the face, so it is worth paying special attention to their care. The first step to beauty is cleanliness. Fresh lemon is used as a hand cleanser all over India. In restaurants an Indian meal is brought to a close with the waiter bringing a silver finger bowl of warm water with a slice of lemon floating in it. Acidic and fragrant, it removes stains and even banishes all the oil and aroma of curry, leaving the hands fresh and clean. Some women rub oil and granulated sugar on their hands to clean them, then rinse with warm water and dry the hands gently. Salt may be substituted for sugar if the hands are particularly gritty.

deep cleanser for hands

i tsp clear honey

I egg white

I tsp glycerine

2 tsp oatmeal

Mix all the ingredients together to form a paste and apply liberally to the hands, especially to areas that are discoloured. Leave the mixture on for thirty minutes, then rinse.

glycerine cuticle softener

I tbsp castor oil

I tbsp glycerine

Mix the ingredients together well and apply to the cuticles. Leave for half an hour and then rinse off. Dry the hands and apply hand cream.

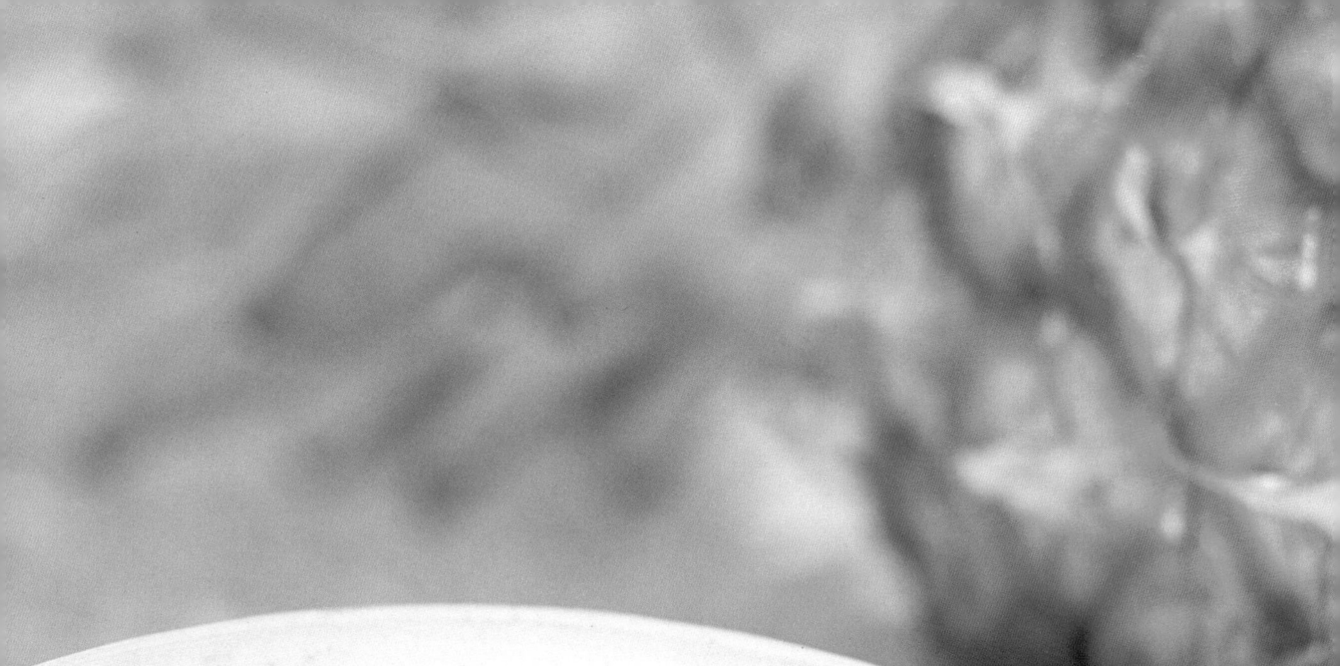

fruity cuticle softener (THIS PAGE)

This preparation works equally well for the feet. Fresh pineapple contains citric and malic acids which clean the cuticles. It also contains a ferment called bromeline, which acts as a softener. The enzymes of papaya are known for their tenderising properties and in fact papaya is used extensively in Indian cookery to soften meat for curries. The egg yolk provides silky protein for conditioning; whereas the cider vinegar, with its gentle acidic quality, cleans the cuticles.

1 tbsp fresh pineapple or papaya juice

¼ tsp egg yolk

1 tsp cider vinegar

Blend all the ingredients well and apply to the cuticles. Leave for half an hour and wash off.

Over-exposure to harsh detergents makes the hands and nails dry and sensitive. Mix together equal quantities of rosewater and glycerine and smooth in to repair any damage. Glycerine is extracted commercially from fats and has restorative properties. A deliciously fragrant mixture of honey and orange juice also softens battered hands and any leftovers can be used as a face mask for refining the complexion. The reverse also applies: use leftover face mask on your hands to condition them.

The most effective way to soften rough hands is to soak them in a shallow basin of olive oil for ten minutes. Massage the oil into the hands and pat off the excess. Do this every night for a week and see the difference for yourself. Also try this luxurious recipe…

rich hand cream

1 egg white

½ cup white wax

½ cup almond oil

pinch of alum

Blend all the ingredients together with a wooden spoon till a smooth cream is formed. Store this in a glass jar and use daily. The alum in this preperation prevents the egg white from curdling during the vigorous mixing process and helps keep the cream fresh longer. It is available

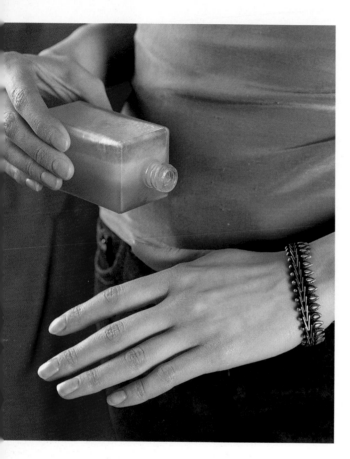

gradually into the honey mixture. Keep whisking until the mixture cools. Store in a glass bottle and use daily.

nail care

Beautifully shaped, glowing nails of even length add grace to the hands. They need only a few coats of nail varnish to achieve a highly glamourous and sophisticated look.

Nails are made of keratin, a sort of dead protein, that, when abused, is liable to split and break. Harsh detergents, the wrong diet, and growing them too long all have a weakening effect. Shorter nails are stronger because, if over-long, they grow away from their point of anchorage to the nail bed at the cuticle and tend to snap at the slightest pressure. The cuticle seals the space between the nail and its bed, preventing dirt and bacteria entering it and causing infection. That is why it is extremely unwise to clip the cuticles. If you have folds of skin that look like over-grown cuticles, have them attended to by a professional manicurist.

Brittle nails are almost always a result of specific mineral or vitamin deficiencies and calcium-rich foods such as milk should help. For intensive treatment take a calcium tablet before going to bed. It will strengthen the nails and, being a mild tranquilliser, will help you fall asleep as well. Zinc is also required to keep the nails free of white spots, so seafood lovers can have the time of their life fortifying their nails – oysters are a particularly good source. Brewer's yeast is another good source of zinc. The spots do tend to grow out with the nail and by eating a good diet you should be able to stop new ones from appearing.

Nail varnish remover contains acetone, a powerful solvent, that will dissolve even some plastics and rubber. It

from Indian shops. White wax is available from health and art shops (it is also used for batik).

honey hand lotion (ABOVE)

1 tsp clear honey

2 tbsp almond oil

4 tbsp rosewater

1 tsp cider vinegar

Warm the honey and then whisk with the almond oil. Warm the rosewater and cider vinegar and beat them is extremely drying and over-use of nail varnishes (which also contain some harmful chemicals) and removers will make the nails brittle and discolour them. Leave nails bare as much as you possibly can.

One of the recipes handed down to me by my grandmother Sushila was for this nail strengthener. When I was a little girl my grandmother stored this cream in a beautiful, blue glass bottle on her dressing table. The faceted stopper of the bottle would cast a million prismatic rainbows in the early morning sunshine and this would often be the first thing I would see on waking up in her bed.

Sushila's nail strengthener

1 tbsp anhydrous lanolin

1 tsp iodine

Put the lanolin in a heat-proof bowl placed over a pan of water and heat gently until melted. Mix in the iodine and stir until well blended. Cool slightly and pour into a bottle. Apply a tiny amount and let it work on the cuticles and nails overnight.

anti-nail-bite remedy

Here is my grandmother's cure for nail-biting; it uses bitter gourd, a long, ridged, bright green vegetable available at all Indian grocers.

1 bitter gourd (karela)

½ tsp salt

Chop the gourd roughly and sprinkle with salt. Allow it to stand till the juice runs, then collect this and paint on to the nails. The acutely bitter taste will make sure that you leave your nails well alone!

a manicure

Manicures are important for the upkeep of the hands and good circulation in the hands is essential to maintain their flexibility. Start your manicure by boosting circulation with the following exercises that even very young girls do as a part of their initial training in Indian classical dance. Do each exercise a couple of times:

1 Clench both fists tightly, hold for a moment and then stretch the fingers out as wide as possible till you feel them tingling.

2 Keeping the hands limp, rotate them at the wrist, first clockwise then anti-clockwise.

3 Curl the fingers in one at a time, starting from the little finger and ending with the thumb. Reach for your wrist with each of your fingers and then close with the thumb.

4 Gently pull each finger outwards with the other hand.

5 Link the fingers of both hands and bring the wrists together, Now, open out the hands, keeping the wrists together, and stretching the fingers as much as possible.

6 Join the fingertips then spread the fingers wide, opening the palm as if you are showing someone five fingers. Do this rapidly like 'twinkling stars' at least five times.

now for the outside...

1 File the nails gently (cutting can weaken nails or cause them to split). Aim for a rounded tip so that the nail, from base to tip, is oval in shape.

2 Soak the hands in a shallow bowl of warm water. You can, if you wish, add a spoonful of herbal shampoo.

3 Gently pat the hands dry and massage cuticle softener cream (see pages 76–7) into the cuticles.

4 Gently push back the cuticles with the tip of an orange

stick wrapped in cotton wool, keeping in mind the oval shape of the nail.

5 Use a small nail brush dipped in the sudsy water to clean the nails, taking care to work away dirt from underneath and around the edges. Dry the hands.

6 Now massage the hands with a good moisturising cream (see page 38), making small circles on the palm and the back of each hand and by rubbing the palms together and wringing the hands. Continue for five to ten minutes.

7 Soak the hands in warm water for a minute, cleaning under the nails as well, and pat dry. Make sure that the nails are free from grease or the varnish will not 'catch'.

8 Now apply your favourite nail varnish in smooth strokes from base to tip. Apply two to three coats for best colour results. You can also use a base coat to protect the nails and a top coat to seal the varnish. Remember to leave the nails nude for a few days between applications of varnish so that they can 'breathe'.

care of the feet

We seldom realise how much hard work our feet do for us and we owe it to them to look after them so that they remain pretty and healthy for a long time.

coconut heel soother

The southern state of Kerala is richly dotted with coconut trees. The women here are known for their polished skin and ebony hair, which is the good work of pure coconut oil. This oil has marvellous softening and restorative properties. Rub a tiny amount into your heels at bedtime. Alternatively, try the following heel soother. Chickpea

flour, being a good skin polisher will smooth the skin while the coconut milk nourishes it.

3 tbsp coconut milk

1 tsp chickpea flour

Blend the ingredients together to form a fine paste and apply to the heels. Leave on for 15 minutes and rinse off.

foot problems

In the past, walking around barefoot must surely have brought along its own problems and our ancestors had to find answers from the natural resources around them. Today corns and callouses are more the result of uncomfortable and ill-fitting footwear than anything else.

CORNS If you have corns try one of the remedies below. Rub a thick slice of fresh garlic on the corn and, if possible, tie the slice to the corn with a plaster when you go to bed. Garlic juice boosts the circulation and promotes healing. A slice of fresh tomato or pineapple (the acids in both are helpful) tied to a corn will also soften it.

A poultice of ivy leaves soaked in vinegar is a western home remedy for corns, the Indian equivalent is to crush fresh marigold leaves and apply the juice nightly to corns.

My aunt Revati had a sure-fire cure for my uncle's persistent corns – she would tie a piece of soft muslin (you can use cotton) soaked in turpentine oil over them and leave it on overnight. She also sat him down with his feet in a tub of warm water and bicarbonate of soda and, if I remember rightly, gave him the household accounts to write in the meantime!

cool balm for corns

1 cup coconut oil

2 tbsp oil of camphor

1 tbsp oil of turpentine

Coconut oil tends to set in cold weather. Melt it if necessary, then beat in the other ingredients until the mixture cools. Put into a jar and allow to set (you can put it in the fridge in summer). Rub a little on to corns twice a day.

hard or calloused soles

Wearing the wrong footwear or straining the feet excessively can result in hard skin on the soles or heels with tiny, deep grooves.

A common complaint suffered by Indian women is 'cracked' heels due to exposure to the elements and dust – unavoidable in view of the open, summery footwear they have to use for comfort. The answer is available from countless street vendors who sell all shapes and colours of pumice stones for a few rupees each. Natural pumice stones are available all over the world and are infinitely safer for removing hard skin than harsh metal scourers, which can tear the skin.

Vimla's foot bath

When I was a teenager, my classical dance training meant eight-hour practice sessions at weekends. Sunday night always saw me sitting with my feet soaking in my mother Vimla's

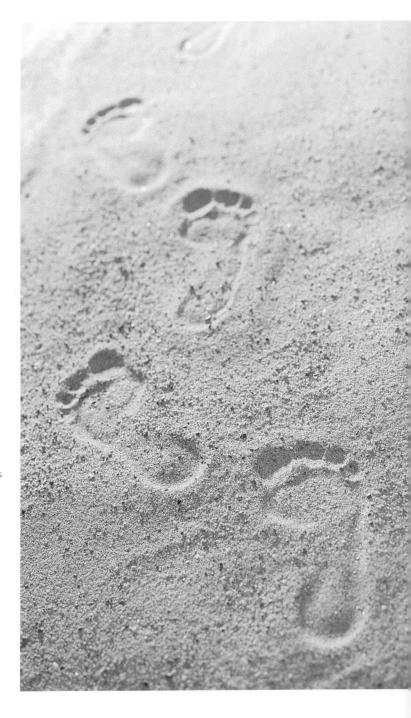

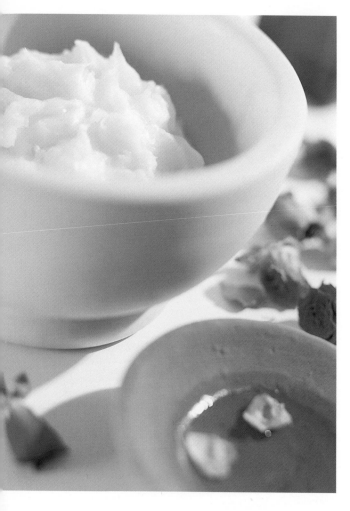

coco-rose foot cream (LEFT)

Around the seaside of southern India women rub callouses on the feet with a pumice stone and follow this with a massage with kokum butter. Kokum is a fruit native to coastal India, but the butter can be bought in Indian shops worldwide. If you can't find it, try this recipe.

½ cup coconut oil

I tsp glycerine

2 tbsp rosewater

Put all the ingredients into a screw-top jar and shake well as you would for a salad dressing. Apply at bedtime and protect the feet with cotton socks.

treatment for sore feet

According to Ayurveda, the live bacteria in the yoghurt have excellent healing properties. Vinegar has been traditionally used to treat bruises and sores.

2 tbsp plain live yoghurt

I tsp vinegar

Mix the ingredients together and brush on to the feet.

remedy for tired feet. Salt and clove oil boost the circulation and castor oil softens hard skin on the heels and soles.

handful of sea salt

5 drops clove oil

I tbsp castor oil

Mix all the ingredients in a shallow bowl of warm water and soak the feet until the water is cold.

a pedicure

Precede your pedicure with some exercises for the feet. Do each one five times unless otherwise stated.

I Point your toes, then flex your feet.

2 Rotate the foot from the ankle, first clockwise and then anti-clockwise.

3 Pull each toe gently, then squeeze the toes together with your hand. Do this a couple of times.

4 Walk on your toes for a count of ten, then on your heels for another ten.

It is also very relaxing to literally 'put your feet up' after a hard day. In India a massage at the end of the day is normal for many people. In the villages a massage-wallah kneads away tiredness from the back, legs and feet of wealthy men as they relax in the open under an umbrella of stars.

now for the outside...

1 Remove all traces of nail varnish.

2 Soak your feet in warm, soapy water and relax for ten minutes.

3 Gently rub a pumice stone all over the feet, paying attention to the heels and soles of the feet. You could use a foot scourer though this can be too abrasive.

4 File the nails straight across and even out rough edges.

5 Remove dirt from under and around the nails and brush the whole foot gently with a foot brush.

6 Dry the feet with a soft towel, taking particular care between the toes.

7 Apply cuticle cream (see pages 76–7) or oil around the toe nails and massage well.

8 Push back the cuticles with an orange stick wrapped in cotton wool.

9 Wipe the nails and apply foot cream or moisturiser (see page 38) . Massage well for ten minutes.

10 Immerse the feet in warm water again for just a minute. Dry them and wipe the nails well to ready them for nail varnish. Apply the varnish in three strokes, and separate the toes with balls of cotton wool to avoid smudging.

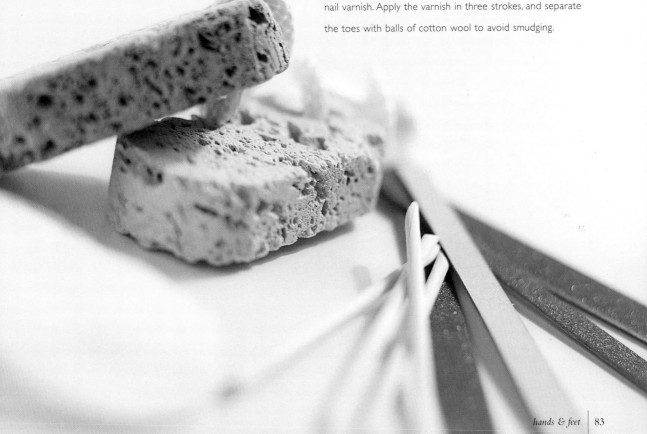

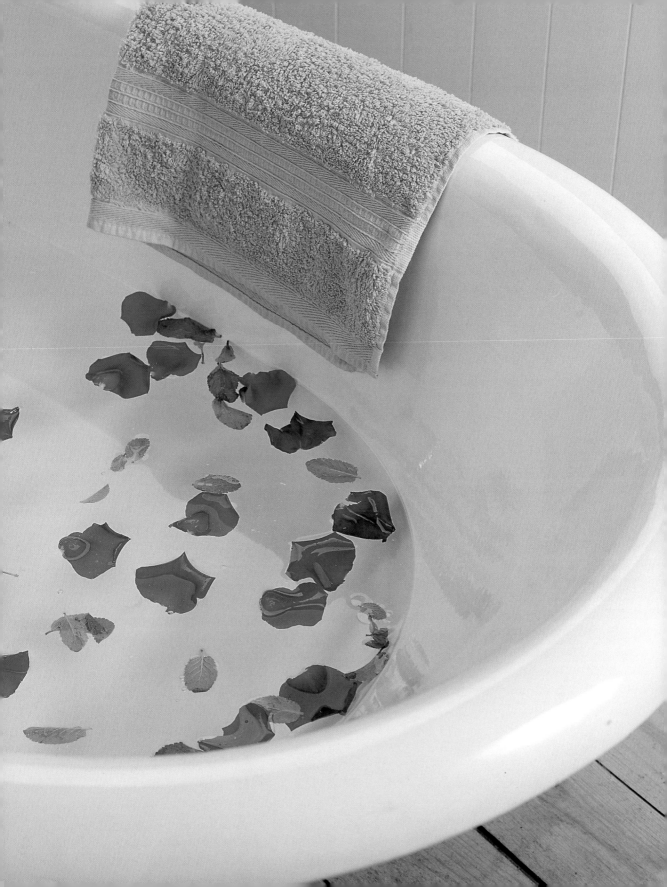

'Her shapely, youthful figure is draped with the garment of a starry sky, her earrings have bunches of pearls like celestial constellations and the scent of her burnished body, like that of a musk deer, fills the air.'

hymn to the goddess Durga

hygiene & perfume

The first deity to be worshipped in a Hindu home is the elephant-headed, pot-bellied god of wisdom, Ganesha. The legend narrating his birth has become a bedtime story in many Indian homes. Ganesha is the second son of Lord Shiva and his wife, the goddess Parvati. The story goes that one day, as Parvati was entering her bath-chamber, she realised that there was no one to guard her door. She playfully collected the unwashed but divinely perfumed, outermost layer of skin from her body and created a young boy, Ganesha, who would be completely loyal to her. Smiling at her new creation, she asked him not to allow anyone in. She then went inside to bathe, leaving fearless little Ganesha outside. A while later her husband Shiva came along with his army of followers and, on being refused entry and not being able to recognise this new boy, became so angry that he ordered his devotees to chop off

his head. Shortly afterwards Parvati came out, fragrant and refreshed. She could not believe her eyes when she saw Ganesha lying in a pool of blood. Shiva realised his mistake and begged for forgiveness, but she was inconsolable. That is why Shiva sent his followers to bring back the head of the first living being they saw. This happened to be an elephant and that is how Ganesha, created out of his mother's perfume but who, in a more philosophical light, represents the dichotomies in each of us (he is greedy but very wise; he is fat but a wonderful dancer), got his elephant's head.

In India, the body is considered to be a temple, a shelter in which resides the Truth of the Cosmos and the spark of Divine Energy. The body is revered and special care is taken of it internally and externally to make it a fit haven for God. Hindus believe that the physical frame confines the soul with onion-like layers of body, mind and intellect and it should therefore be disciplined and clean. The body itself is made up of the five elements, the *pancha-bhuta*, namely water, fire, earth, air and ether. On death they resolve to their initial state. The bodies of great people are believed to have a golden aura of pure light and all divine beings, including saints, are depicted with this glowing halo.

In Hinduism great importance is attached to a bath, which becomes a ritual not only of physical cleansing but also of spiritual sanctity. In the architecture of early Indian civilisations such as Mohenjo Daro and Harrappa, around 2500–1500 BC, rectangular bathing tanks were sited in town centres. Communal baths were the norm and such pools were built to emphasise the beliefs that a ceremonial bath connects the bather with heaven through the medium of water. The tank had steps leading down into the water to ease the bather into a transitional place suspended between several realms. Bathers were supposed to leave their cares behind as they descended into a divine world.

Everywhere in the world certain kinds of water are considered healing and spas have been established at places

where such water occurs naturally. In many places in India in Vajreshwari near Mumbai or in Himachal Pradesh, for example – natural hot-water springs with optimum amounts of sulphuric compounds, proved to be beneficial to the skin, simmer under the surface of the earth and flow out with a bubbling energy. This natural mineral water is channelled into bathing rooms where patrons enjoy a communal dip. Patients of skin ailments are taken to these hot springs for a recuperative bath.

Early Hindu scriptures such as the *Vedas* (c. 1500–900 BC) suggest the best way of having *snana* or a ritual bath. The rules of the Vastu-Shastra, an ancient text about the dos and don'ts of home construction and design, declare that a bathroom must face the east to catch the rays of the early-morning sun. The sun is said to suffuse the body with power and energy. The ritual bath began with *majjana* or immersing the entire body in water, followed by *achamana* or rinsing of the mouth. *Padya* was the washing of the feet and *abhisheka* or anointing with various liquids such as oil, yoghurt, milk and honey came next. *Kshala* was the pouring of water over the body, *dhavala* the rubbing to remove dirt and, finally, *marjana* the wiping of the body to dry it.

Ritual baths are still performed by Hindus all over the country at auspicious times. For instance, a special bath is taken by traditional students of the *Vedas* and of Sanskrit at the end of their studies. This washes away the aura of celibacy, and therefore sanctity, that they have collected through their studentship and makes them ready to join social life as householders. In the Hindu marriage ceremony both the bride and the groom are given a ceremonial bath with turmeric (considered by Ayurveda to be cleansing and antiseptic) and fresh cream, after which they are not allowed to leave the house until the wedding. Temple deities made of stone are also given a daily bath with *panchamrit*, a mixture of honey, sugar, ghee (clarified butter), yoghurt and milk, as a form of worship. The gods are then anointed with fragrant sandalwood, dressed in silks and jewels and presented to the public.

The festival of Diwali at the beginning of winter brings a spectacle of lights and fireworks. A Hindu family wakes at dawn and, after the symbolic destroying of evil in the form of a small, bitter fruit called *kareet* which is crushed, everyone has a ritual bath of oil and *ubtan*, a fragrant mixture of sandalwood and other herbs. Only after this bath and prayers does the family sit down to a sumptuous diwali breakfast.

People all over the world value perfume, and perfumery has become an intricate science. In Vedic times, as today, nature provided fragrance and it was the Mughals, who invaded India around six centuries ago, who gave perfume its glamour in this country. They refined the process of distilling fragrances from flowers, leaves and bark and called it *ittar* or *attar*. *Attar*, a strong, concentrated perfume, is available even today. A variety of scents such as rose, jasmine and sandalwood, as well as Indian florals such as *mogra*, *saayli*, *chameli* and *juhi*, are bottled in tiny crystal jars and line the shelves of small, Mughal-influenced perfume shops.

For most career women today a daily bath means a quick shower to get clean. But there is more to a bath than that. For every woman the bath is where her beauty routine begins. The word 'bath' itself conjures up images of relaxation and pampering and, depending on the time of day, a bath should be relaxing or stimulating. The Mughal

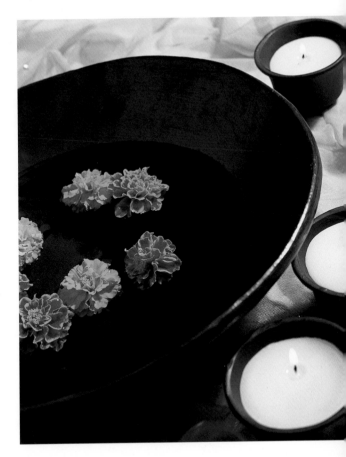

A well-known herbalist and beautician in New Delhi recommends a special bath once a week. She suggests throwing a handful of fragrant rose or marigold petals along with a teaspoonful of almond oil into the bath and soaking yourself for half an hour with nothing on your mind except your dreams. According to her, this bath revitalises you for the hectic week ahead.

baths to soak

Every Indian girl is taught that a daily bath is vital for her cleanliness and beauty. In many south Indian homes the woman of the house rises before dawn to have a cleansing bath before she enters the kitchen to prepare the day's meal – so ingrained is the concept of purity. It is considered a sacrilege to enter a place of worship without having bathed. Indian women do not, however, look upon a bath as merely cleansing: it is also the ultimate luxury.

The bathroom should be your pleasure room – full of secret delights and treats. It is very difficult to feel beautiful in an unattractive, dimly lit room, which demands a quick exit. Instead choose plants that thrive in a steamy environment, twinkling lamps that cast a glow, scented candles that suffuse the senses and bathroom accessories that are designed to pamper.

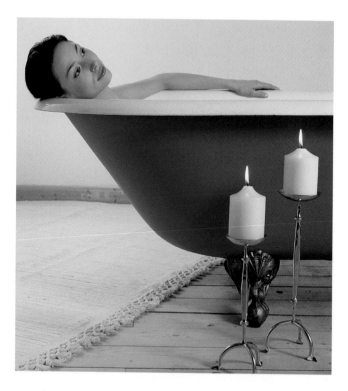

above
Bathtime is time to yourself – a private time to play out the fantasies in your mind and spoil yourself. A good bath should leave you feeling refreshed in body and in spirit.

queens of India were famed for their fresh milk baths – which do not leave the skin sticky or smelly as you might expect. On the contrary, the protein in the milk makes the skin satin-smooth and glowing. Even today a good skin-firming bath is prepared simply by mixing a heaped teaspoonful of milk powder or a cup of fresh milk along with a teaspoonful of oatmeal into warm water. The ambience that was created for the queens is also easy to copy today. Candles scented with relaxing perfumes like rose or lavender, soft music and your favourite drink will instantly soothe the body and mind.

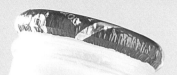

The erstwhile Maharajas made exotic bathing an art form. 'Teak trunks for five of the wives of the Maharaja of Patiala were simple enough, each one lined in blue velvet fitted with solid silver wash-bowls, soap dishes, hand basins and toothbrush holders. The bottles for pouring hot water had tiger head spouts and the "goesunders", the coyly named chamber pots, in one-eighth inch silver,' writes Ann Morrow in *Highness — the Maharajas of India*. The women of the royal household would meet each morning beside beautiful, lotus-shaped, marble baths and have their bodies anointed by handmaidens with sandalwood and cream. These rose-strewn pools became the playgrounds of the lovely maharanis.

In their book *Lives of the Indian Princes* Charles Allen and Sharada Dwivedi describe the luxury of such a bath: 'In Travancore this occupied the first two hours of the Maharani's day. We used no soap in those days. Instead there were three silver bowls, each with a different oil for the face, the body and the hair and four copper vessels filled with four kinds of herbal waters. Your hair was washed first using green "thali" paste made from freshly plucked leaves, then washed and oiled with coconut oil and dried with a thin porous material called "tortu". Then your body was washed, powdered gram (chickpeas) was applied and removed with a circular sort of sponge called "incha" made from a fibrous bark and you were washed again with "Nalpamaravellam" water, absolutely red in colour and made by boiling the bark of forty different trees.'

Alas, it is not possible for all of us to bathe in sparkling silver bathtubs while attendants fulfil our every wish, but here are some baths to soak in that will make your skin glow and your mood as insouciant as that of a queen.

rose bath oil

The almond oil is especially good for dry skins. The addition of a little shampoo helps to keep the oil from sticking to the bath and lets it cling to the skin instead.

1 cup almond oil

2 tbsp shampoo

4 tbsp rosewater

fragrant rose petals (optional)

Whisk together all the ingredients till well blended and bottle. Pour a little of this oil into a warm bath. If you wish, sprinkle a few fragrant rose petals on top and enjoy!

As an alternative to the rose bath oil, you can simply add a few drops of a relaxing, fragrant oil such as orange or lemon or a stimulating one such as cardamom or basil to your bath.

refreshing bath
A tablespoonful of Epsom salts, sea salt crystals or even ordinary table salt stirred into a hot bath will revive the body by taking away fatigue, aches and pains. A salt bath is especially welcome after a hard day at work.

milk bath
The luxurious feeling of floating in a white cloud is easily achieved by making yourself a simple milk bath. Milk is full of goodness — it contains protein that is vital to skin and it tightens, whitens and soothes the skin. Even pouring a pint of milk into the bath will make a difference, but for real extravagance tie a cupful of milk powder in a cloth sachet and slowly rub over your body so that the water becomes milky gradually. If you would rather shower, make a thick paste of milk powder and water and apply to the skin. Leave it on for 10–15 minutes to make your skin feel like satin.

winter bath When the weather outside is blustery or snowy and you feel shivers prance over your skin, a mustard bath will leave you feeling warm and toasty. Mix a tablespoonful of mustard powder with a little water and add the paste to your bath. If you prefer showering, you can massage your body with the mustard paste. Women in Punjab have a weekly mustard bath. The Punjabi winter is cold and misty and in December the countryside seems covered with carpets of gold as the cool breeze ripples through endless mustard fields.

herb bath A handful of herbs in the bath water will add fragrance and heal and smooth the skin. Particularly good are marigold petals or leaves, mint leaves (really refreshing too!), orange and lemon peel or basil leaves. You can also indulge yourself by throwing in your favourite flowers: try those that are easily available such as freesias (my favourite), chrysanthemums or sweet peas.

soda bath Anyone who has been in the sun too long will know the distress of burnt, peeling skin. Adding to your bath a few teaspoonfuls of bicarbonate of soda, which is alkaline and easily available, will soothe skin that is red and irritated.

starch bath My friend Alka always says that her lovely, even-toned skin is wholly due to the starch baths she was given as a young girl. Her mother would simply grate a raw potato and put it into a muslin pouch to rub over young Alka's body. Many Indian women also use the starchy water that is left over from the daily cooking of rice as a body wash. This rice water sets into a gel when cold and can be massaged on to the body like soap. Starch has a softening and whitening effect on the skin and also soothes and relieves tension.

vinegar Vinegar has the dual properties of controlling blemishes on an oily skin and nourishing flaky, dry skin. Add a couple of tablespoonfuls to the bath along with a few drops of floral essence to mask the sour, acid smell. A teaspoonful of fresh lemon juice, which is a natural and fragrant lightener, can help to even out unhealthy skin tone.

a wake-up bath Every culture around the world has considered heat to be naturally healing and relaxing. In ancient India sages and yogis would have hot, steamy baths and then dive into icy streams to tone the skin and to get the senses alive and tingling. Today all of Scandinavia enjoys sauna parties based on this principle. For your own 'wake-up', step into a warm bath and massage the body well. Finish with a minute in a shower as cold as you can bear. This bath is sure to 'open' your eyes and kick-start the body for the day's activities.

removal of hair

For some reason every society has expected beautiful women to be smooth-skinned and hairless. While a profusion of hair on the head is appreciated, it is usually considered unattractive elsewhere on the body and something to be removed.

Body hair is normal and not at all unfeminine; although patriarchal conditioning through the ages has us believe otherwise. In India young mothers are taught to massage their baby girl's soft skin gently with chickpea (gram flour) mixed with fresh cream, to rub off any fine down and to hamper later growth of hair on the arms, legs, back and shoulders.

shaving

In India a razor has always been considered a man's property, but these days more and more younger women and teenage girls who wear western-style clothes want to be hair-free all the time and are buying their own shaving razor. Whereas Indian dresses and saris are capable of hiding arms and legs (and see you through the regrowth stage), short skirts and shorts will betray you immediately. Although shaving does not necessarily mean a more abundant re-growth, the hair does appear thicker and more coarse because of the blunt edge that has been sliced by the razor. Shaved arms and legs feel bristly within a couple of days and the procedure has to be repeated every day to be really spot-on. Dry shaving can give you unsightly nicks and cuts, so do take the time to use soap and water, and to work up a really good lather before you put the blade to your skin. Keep your razor absolutely clean and cream the area well afterwards. In-grown hairs can be a problem for shaved legs – a regular, gentle rub with a pumice stone will take care of this.

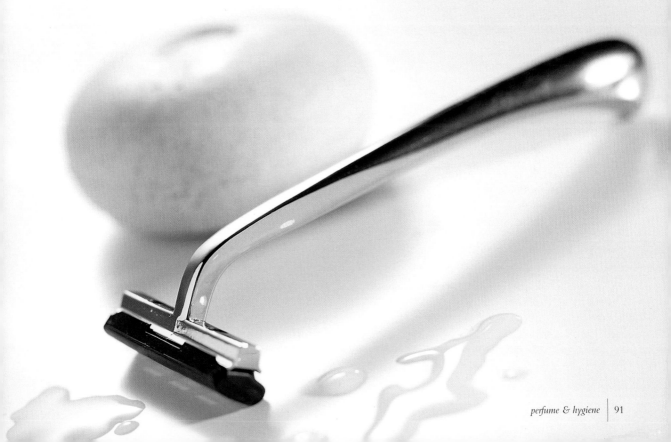

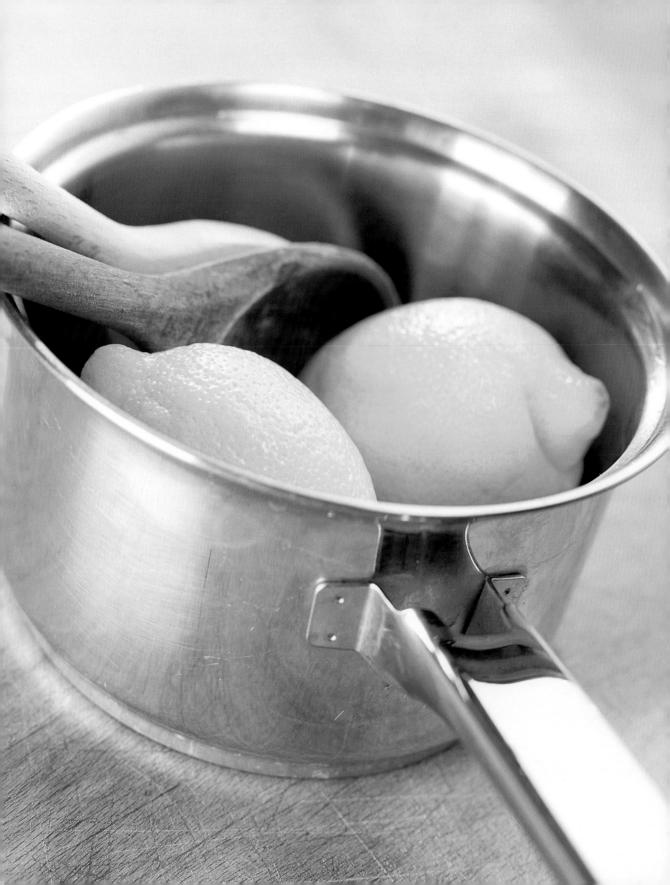

plucking

The easiest way of removing stray hairs on the face, especially around the eyebrows and the chin, is to pluck them out individually with a good pair of tweezers. Wiping the area with astringent or a gentle antiseptic beforehand will remove oil so that tiny hairs can be captured, and after plucking will ensure that the pores close quickly to avoid any infection. Never pull out hairs that are growing from warts or moles – these are best left to professionals.

To remove stray hairs from around the breasts and on the stomach, do not pluck as this can stimulate the root to produce stronger hair; instead cut as close to the skin as possible using a small pair of scissors or, if you do not mind the daily ritual, shave with a razor designed for sensitive skin.

bleaching

Although bleaching does not get rid of hair, it is a wonderfully painless way of disguising any dark hair by lightening it to your skin colour. Bleach can be used on the face, arms, chest, and legs – in fact just about anywhere on the body. Do try a patch test if you have even an inkling of a sensitive skin.

Several good commercial bleaching products are available, but many Indian women still make the following bleaching paste at home with quite successful results.

1 tbsp 20-volume peroxide

enough fuller's earth to make a paste

few drops of ammonia

Mix all the ingredients to a paste and spread on to the required area. Rinse off after 15–20 minutes. You may need to repeat this treatment for darker hairs till they are light and then re-treat less frequently to maintain the look.

A natural bleach such as lemon juice can be spread over the face for half an hour for a mild lightening action.

waxing

Waxing is an age-old method of hair removal and was reportedly used by Indian maharanis even a few hundred years ago. Indian women today far prefer waxing their legs to shaving them. Hair takes longer to regrow (four to six weeks) and, with time, the roots weaken enough to decrease regrowth. In India the wax is prepared at home or by a beautician; it is not available off the shelf.

home-made wax

This recipe makes enough to treat both legs:

4 tbsp sugar

2 tbsp lemon juice

The amount of lemon juice will depend on factors such as the weather, the moisture in the sugar and the amount of heat applied, so do keep extra juice handy. Mix the ingredients and heat over a low heat stirring constantly. As the mixture turns golden, remove from the heat and keep stirring till it thickens. You will need to regulate the heat here – practice will tell you how much. You should aim to get a 'wax' that is the colour and consistency of honey. Although the process may seem bothersome at first, the economy of it set against the cost of visits to a professional salon will help you to persevere. Allow the wax to cool slightly. If it becomes too thick, it will set like caramel, so you need to add a few more drops of lemon juice to dilute it a bit.

left
Fresh lemon juice cooked with sugar makes perfect hair-removing wax while mildly bleaching the skin.

Now you need some strips of thick cotton cloth. Take a little wax on a blunt knife and apply to the treatment area in long strokes in the same direction as the hair grows. Slap on a cloth strip and press down well. Hold the skin taut and pull in one tug in the opposite direction to the growth of the hair. This will be painful at first but you will be surprised at how quickly the skin gets used to the pulling. Continue this, changing the strips as they become layered with wax, until the area is completely free of hair. Home waxing works well on the arms and legs, though under-arms can be frustratingly unreachable (ask a friend to do them) and facial skin is too delicate to be pulled and tugged. You will notice, however, that the sugar and lemon confection conditions the skin, leaving it soft and silky. Commercially made wax is also available in the west and makes a good but more expensive alternative. Waxing, like shaving, sometimes causes in-grown hairs – again, simply rub the area gently with a pumice stone while you are in the bath.

threading

Most of India's city women visit the local beauty parlour on a regular basis. A majority of these salons are run by Chinese families who migrated to India and settled in Calcutta around 1947 when they got wind of a major change in the political system of their native country. They later spread to other parts of the country. The Chinese parlours are instantly distinguishable because of their native Chinese names like King Leong, Ming's Pavilion and Hunan, written in a typical bamboo-stalk font, vying with their Indian cousins which are quaintly called Charms, Silhouette or Figurina.

All these beauty parlours claim that most of their cus- tomers ask for their eyebrows to be 'threaded', a procedure that is popular among all ages and classes of women in India. Threading is simple once you have got the hang of it, but it is infinitely easier to do to someone else rather than to yourself. One end of a cotton thread (the kind used for sewing) is held between the teeth while the middle of the thread is held in a taut loop with one hand and the other end is manoeuvered by the other hand. The mouth and hands work to a rhythm, catching the stray hairs within the loop and plucking them out with the movement of the thread. The procedure is quite similar to the modern hair removal devices that work on electricity.

depilation

Depilatories are creams, gels or spray foams that dissolve the hair below the surface of the skin but do not destroy the root. Regrowth is quite coarse and appears within a week to ten days. Look for specialised products for specific areas, and if using for the first time, try a patch test.

electrolysis

Electrolysis is the only method which promises the possibility of permanent removal, but even so, no one can guarantee that there will not be even the slightest regrowth. A fine needle is inserted into the hair follicle and a low electric current shoots through the hair bulb to destroy it. Once this happens, the hair will never grow again or will become very weak. This procedure is very time-consuming as it needs to be repeated for best results and should be left to professionals. It is usually done on small areas such as the face or on the breasts. With a skilled operator there should be a minimum of pain and no scarring.

body odour

'The fact that the zanana (women's quarters) was officially out of bounds to the male sex did not mean that it was inaccessible to visitors female or male even if the latter might have to conduct their business from the far side of a curtain or chik screen. The visits of traders or sellers of wares were always particularly welcome… the attarwalla (perfume seller) would come…,' recollects Leela Mulgaonkar about daily life in the palaces of India in *Lives of the Indian Princes*.

In the past women may have had to live with body odour at some time in their life: smells of cooking, sweaty work and few washing facilities would all have contributed. Today, with modern plumbing and an array of deodorants available, no woman should smell unpleasant.

One of the greatest luxuries that can be enjoyed by a woman is perfume. It makes you feel positive, sends out messages of allure to those around you and makes a statement about your personality. Imagine the pleasure of pouring a capful of perfumed gel on to a sponge for a body massage, of smoothing on scented body lotion or splashing on cologne…

The first step to being cleanly fragrant is to wear only natural fibres next to the skin. This allows the skin to 'breathe' and sweat to evaporate. Indian cotton is prized for its softness and is always in demand. Regular washing with soap and water will carry off perspiration and neutralise odour for a while. 'Defuzzing' also helps – under-arm hair notoriously traps bacteria that act on perspiration and give rise to a typical, unpleasant smell.

Then comes the ultimate grandeur of perfume. Women have always associated perfume with allure. The marbled bedrooms of

below

An ancient *attar-dani* or perfume casket with traditional glass-stopper bottles of perfume. Only a tiny drop of these strong scented herbal *attars* are used, so they often last several years.

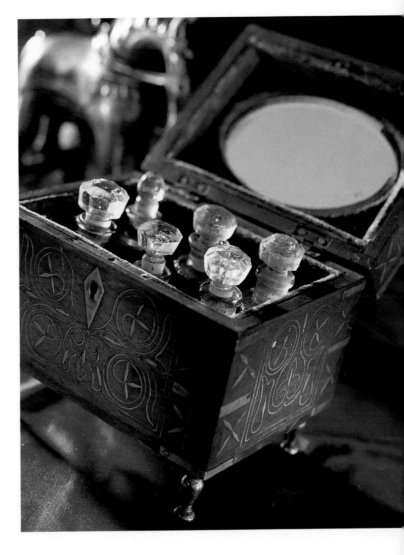

the Mughal queens were reputed to be scented with rose and saffron, creating an ambience of opulence while they rested on fat, gold-embroidered pillows. Cleopatra is said to have perfumed the sails of her barge as she set out to meet Mark Antony. The word perfume means 'through smoke': the earliest perfumes were worn by walking through the smoke of a fire to which scented herbs and spices had been added. Even today fragrant incense is burnt in every Indian temple and many Hindu homes are perfumed with *dhoop*, a pot-pourri of ingredients like camphor and sandalwood, that is burnt and left to smoke. The word perfume itself conjures up visions of romance, extravagance and magic, and every women should be a part of its mystery.

India loves perfume; and even the air is redolent with the scent of cardamom and cloves. Traditional perfumes or *attars* are still made in quantity, the most widely used being rose. This is infinitely precious and correspondingly expensive, 500kg (½ ton) of petals being needed to make 450g (1lb) of *attar*. In Mughal times velvety red roses were especially grown in the royal greenhouses to be made into perfume. Although the rose reigns supreme in the Indian scent kingdom, the *kewra* or screw-pine flower comes a close second, followed by jasmine and *khus*, a highly fragrant grass. *Khus* is even woven into door curtains to perfume the surroundings.

The variety of perfumed products on the market is mind-boggling, but remember that however many rare and costly ingredients go into the making of a perfume, the final and most unique one will be added by your own skin. Body chemistry, the oils, minerals and moisture secreted by the glands beneath the skin's surface as well as the composition of your skin will make a particular fragrance smell different on you than on anyone else. Moreover, when a scent is first applied, the individuality of your skin will make it smell different from how it smells in the bottle, and different again a little while later as it warms ups and reacts with the skin.

It is essential to think of fragrance in a wider context than just from a bottle – scented coat hangers, drawer sachets and room sprays will all contribute to the ambience. Try spraying your ironing board with perfume before you iron your clothes. And once you have opened a bottle, use it on yourself rather than let it evaporate into thin air.

Some women may be especially conscious of body odour during menstruation. Fresh blood does not smell; exposure to air for a length of time changes the odour. Wash often with soap and water and keep away from vaginal deodorants, which are unnecessary. They may at times mask a foul odour, which is one of the most important symptoms of a medical condition. Use only cotton underwear that will allow perspiration and smells to evaporate and try not to wear close-fitting synthetic tights all the time.

Anyone who suffers from smelly feet knows the embarrassment they can cause. Indian women seldom have this problem as their feet are left open to sun and air most of the time. The main victims are people who wear synthetic socks and shoes. Scrupulous and enthusiastic hygiene is the answer: wash the feet well (and often), dry them thoroughly and dust them with fine alum powder, one of the most effective natural deodorants. Adding a teaspoonful of powdered alum to a foot bath or even to your bath water will control odour admirably. Choose leather shoes over plastic or resin as the former allow the feet to 'breathe', and at the end of each day swab your feet with witch-hazel to deodorise them. Try to go barefoot whenever possible.

body cleansers & polishers

'First there was an oil massage of the whole body. Each and every part was massaged by three women. One would hold one hand or leg, another would massage the hand while a third did the back and the massaging was very thorough – very light strokes away from the heart and pressing very hard in the other direction. After the oil massage they used to apply "utne", which was a soft cream made out of almonds freshly ground every Sunday morning,' reminisces a princess about her childhood baths in *Lives of the Indian Princes*.

The Indian bathing tradition has always included exfoliation and polishing of the skin. Legendary queens and courtesans have used the outer hairy coir of a coconut, almond paste or the powdered burnt shells of almonds and walnuts, dried and crushed peels of orange, lemon and pomegranate and an assortment of kitchen flours to keep their skin healthy and glowing like gold.

Natural buffing agents are still used today – women in southern Kerala bathe in natural brooks using coconut husk and medicinal bark, while in other parts of the country certain gourds are quartered and then sun-dried to make porous loofahs that resemble honey-combs. Loofahs puff up in water, turning into natural sponges that, when rubbed on the

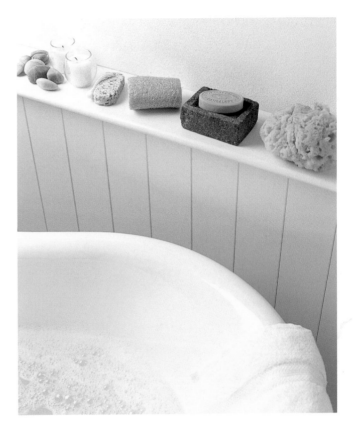

skin in circular movements, slough off dead cells and leave the surface satin-smooth and tingling. In the West a softer version of the loofah is a towelling mitt that is used with soap to lather and cleanse the body. Loofahs and mitts are especially good for areas that are usually overlooked – the back, shoulders and back of the legs. For the most sensitive skin, simply use a sponge; it is less abrasive and will at least freshen the skin without too much friction. Pumice stones are the perfect tools for hard skin on heels and elbows.

above
An assortment of body polishers such as a loofah, pumice stone and a sponge sit on a bath shelf, each offering a tantalising promise of glowing, healthy skin.

a simple skin polisher

Skin polishers give the body a golden glow. Here is one of the easiest you can make at home.

½ cup warm olive oil

½ cup sea salt

Step into the bath and wet your skin all over. Then stand up and dip your hand first into the olive oil and then the salt. Rub the mixture on to your body with gentle, circular movements. You can also use a soft body brush, but your hand will do just as well. Massage your body thoroughly and all over for at least ten minutes. Then rinse off well and towel dry. Your skin will be smooth, soft and glowing.

a traditional skin polisher

This is used by women all over India. The turmeric acts as a natural cleanser and disinfectant and will not turn your skin yellow. The chickpea flour sloughs off dead skin to give unimagined silkiness and the milk will firm up the entire body. Even the tiniest of babies are massaged with this body polisher, but do be careful if you have a history of allergy to wheat or lentil flour – use rice flour instead.

I tablespoon chickpea flour

pinch of turmeric

about 2 tsp of milk

Mix all the the ingredients together and rub on to wet skin instead of soap.

oatmeal body scrub

When the skin is looking especially sallow after a winter of being wrapped up, consider the benefits of an oatmeal scrub. This is wonderfully abrasive and firms up the skin.

2 tbsp oatmeal, barleymeal or even cornflour

water or milk to mix

Mix the oatmeal, barleymeal or cornflour to a paste with the water or milk. Rub the mixture on to the body using gentle, circular movements for two to three minutes. Leave on for a couple more minutes, then rinse off.

fruity skin revitalisers

Massaging the body with a slice of a juicy fruit such as pineapple, mango, papaya or grape will revitalise the skin and add extra glamour to your bathtime. If these fruits are not readily available, oranges, peaches or strawberries will do marvellously. Strawberry juice has long been known to calm rashes and neutralise oily, blemished skin. Imagine the pure luxury of a fresh strawberry bath!

safe tanning

In India we are forever exposed to the dangers associated with tanning because of the tropical sun, notwithstanding the natural melanin in our skin that can cope with it. I am constantly surprised by the universal attitude

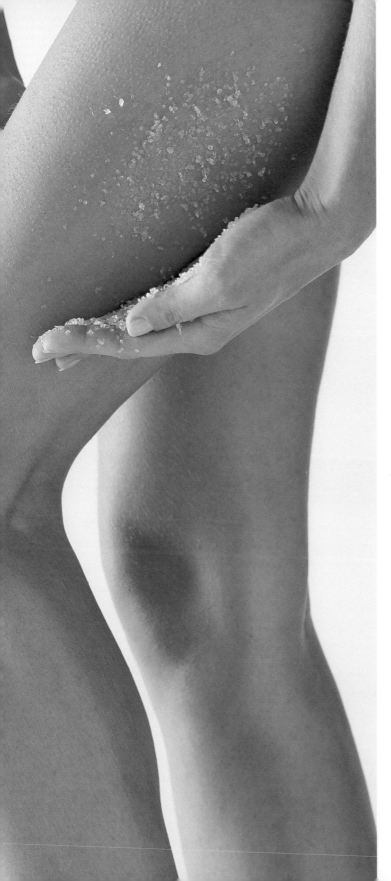

of looking down on 'coloured' people when most of the 'non-coloured' people, irrespective of the proven dangers of excess sun, flock to the world's sunny beaches to acquire a darker colour than their own! There is something attractive about being tanned; people always say it makes them look and feel healthy, but the skin must never be allowed to burn. This is easy to forget when you are on holiday – the liberation of a blue sky overhead and miles of dazzling sea can make you reckless and encourage you to throw caution to the wind.

The rule is that when you want to get brown, you run the risk of burning and therefore you must protect yourself. The culprits that cause the skin to turn red, blister and finally peel are the ultraviolet rays in sunshine and it is these particularly that you need to guard yourself against. The darker your skin, the more capable it will be of withstanding the sun and the less it will burn. Good sense tells us that sunbathing should be done in short bursts and never in the glare of the hot midday sun. Be careful not to fall asleep in the sun – you might wake up looking like a lobster and the pain that follows will eliminate all thoughts of a lovely holiday. If your skin feels hot, pink or sore, you can assume that this particular bout of tanning went on for too

this page
Skin polishers slough off dead skin
leaving the body soft and glowing.

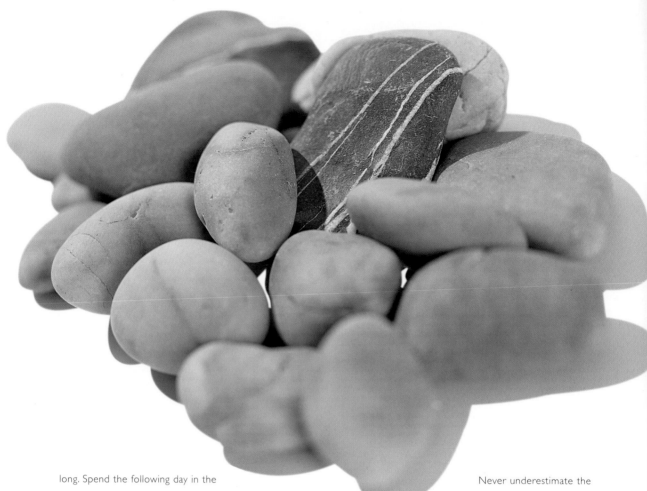

long. Spend the following day in the shade and on the next one take the sun in small doses. If you are going from, say, London to the Mediterranean for a holiday, it is a good idea to acclimatise your skin to ultraviolet light before you go. Make the most of evening or weekend sunshine, however weak, or use your lunch hour to take a walk in the sun so that acquiring a tan on holiday is faster and therefore safer. Everyone has an 'ultimate tan point' beyond which they cannot go without the skin becoming dry and patchy. Doctors have long warned people against prolonged sun tanning because of the serious risks involved, including the possibility of skin cancer. Years and years of drying out the skin in the sun ages it and invites early wrinkles.

Never underestimate the value of a good sunblock cream or lotion. Simple oil is lubricating but will provide no protection at all; instead it will probably only help to fry the skin further. What you need is a lotion, gel or cream with a SPF (sun protection factor) that will protect the skin: follow the instructions on the bottle with great care. Remember, though, that sunblock preparations are not a guarantee against the sun's harmful effects and you need to abide by all the rules of safe tanning. Be sure also to drink plenty of water to prevent dehydration. As soon as you return indoors cool down the body with a tepid bath and oil yourself well to keep the skin supple.

For as long as I can remember, my grandmother has

advocated a cooling mixture of chilled yoghurt and rosewater, mixed in the proportion of a cupful to two tablespoons, as a remedy for sunburn. She would make up quantities of this creamy mixture for us after school picnics, sit us on low stools in the bathroom and bathe us in it from head to toe. A finishing rinse of cool water ensured that we were all set for school the next day. In the west rosewater can easily be substituted with elderflower water, which is equally soothing. A local application of cool Indian tea on affected areas will also bring relief to sunburnt patches. Sunburnt skin will definitely peel, so keep it lubricated with olive or coconut oil fortified with a few drops of vitamin E oil, which is healing.

cucumber cooler for sunburn (RIGHT)

I cup mashed cucumber

I tsp glycerine

Mix together the cucumber and glycerine and refrigerate until chilled. Apply to the affected parts and rinse off after half an hour. Use up this recipe quickly as it will not keep for more than a day.

lemon lotion for burnt skin

2 tbsp lemon juice

I egg white

Whisk the ingredients together until well blended. Put into a pan over low heat and keep stirring until the mixture thickens. Apply to areas that are burnt and leave on; rinsing off is not necessary. Use up within a day.

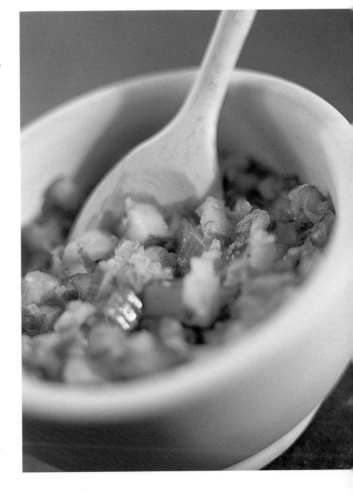

rose lotion

2 tbsp olive oil

2 tbsp glycerine

2 tbsp rosewater

2 tbsp witch-hazel

Shake all the ingredients together in a bottle and refrigerate until cold. Use on skin that is burnt by the sun or by snow 'glare'.

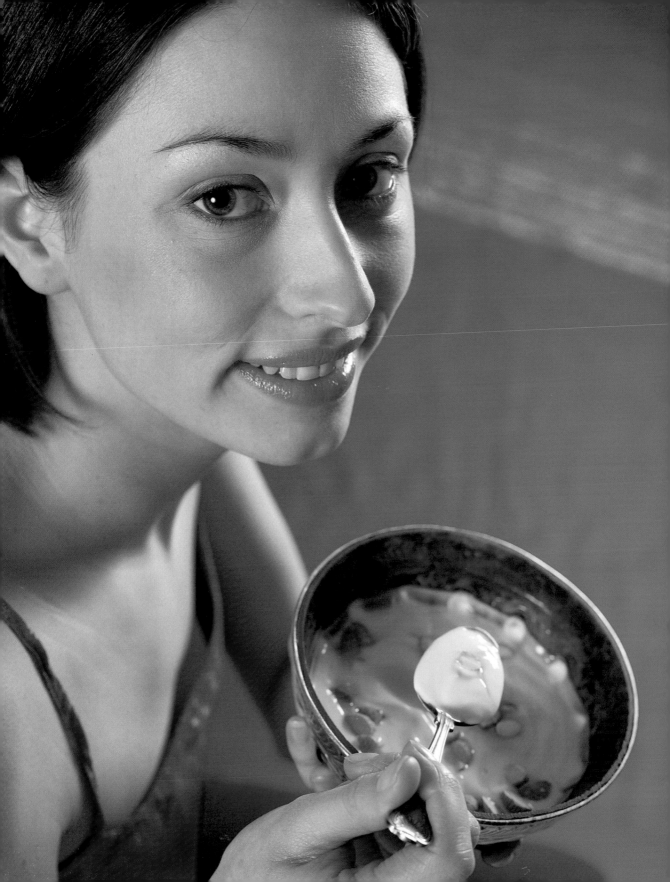

'Her breasts shaped like lotus buds are full like ripe melons, and so close together that there is hardly room between them for a lotus stalk. Her nipples are like the berry of the *kanjidruma*, inviting the lover's teeth.' *Anonymous Sanskrit poem, probably a few centuries old*

body awareness

One of the many words in Sanskrit for woman is *angana*, which means 'having a body'. A few thousand years ago *Stritantra* or female lore was a subject of study with special emphasis on a woman's physical body. The girl child was considered mystical because of her magical ability to reproduce in later life and was classified according to her age and physical development. *Nagnika* was a nude girl under five years of age; *vasu*, clothed at five years; *gauri*, white at the age of six; *vatsa* a calf at seven; *kanya* a maiden at puberty; *lagnika*, ready for marriage; *kishori* in her teens; and *proudha* entering her twenties.

Writers of mythology also contributed their concepts to female lore and divided women into four categories for the purpose of describing them in stories:

1 *Padmini* was a lotus woman, refined and graceful, rounded in breasts and hips and sweet smelling like a lotus.

2 *Chitrini* was like a painting, slim, sensual and fiery.

3 *Shankhini* had a conch-shaped physique and was usually a courtesan who offered all kinds of sexual delights. She was not a home-maker; instead she lived a life of abandon.

4 *Hastini* was an elephant of a woman, graceful, generous and with an abundance of curves that pleased her partners.

These descriptions also appear in the *Kamasutra* of Vatsyayan, affirming the fact that men have always been preoccupied with women. In early mythology, nymphs called *apsaras* were created to be the ideals of beauty and to set up yardsticks against which mortal women were compared for thousands of years thereafter. In the West too female icons have been created and celebrated, from Cranach's Venus in medieval times to the twentieth century's Marilyn Monroe. These have established ideals of perfect beauty that women aspire to even today. Of course these archetypes could be created only in a patri-archal, male-dominated world. Thus in mythology women were depicted as half-dressed creatures who were made for the pleasure of the gods or to seduce and distract those who became a threat to them. In all societies ideals of femininity were placed on a pedestal and other women were expected to try to emulate them.

These ideals and standards have survived the test of time. The world still believes in the power of a woman whose beauty can inspire awe and devotion. There is a dichotomy of belief, however: women everywhere are considered slightly less than men, but they are also worshipped. The women of today, successful in everything they put their mind to, have made it amply clear that beauty and sensuality or power and intelligence in a woman are not mutually exclusive.

In India a woman considers her body to be sacrosanct and the virtues of modesty and chastity are cherished. Exposure of the female form is frowned upon, although the ancient sculptures, modern Hindi films (which are the nation's passion) as well as the ubiquitous female dress, the *sari*, all celebrate and exploit feminine curves to the full! Girls are brought up to believe that romance and sex follow after marriage, which is usually arranged when they are between eighteen and twenty-three years of age. No self-respecting Indian woman will admit to pre-marital affairs as virginity is expected and demanded of her until her wedding day. Today's girl is still comfortable living and working within the parameters laid down by society, which really do not conflict with her sense of identity and personal development.

An Indian girl becomes an entity to guard, nurture and cherish from the day she begins to menstruate. Ayurveda called this *rajas* or the physical sign that a girl was now mature and able to bear children. A woman was segregated during her periods: she retired to a special room, was given certain foods to eat, did not touch anyone including her own children and washed her hair only on the fourth day. After her flow had stopped, she had a ritual cleansing bath. The earliest reason for this practice was that a woman's resistance was considered at its lowest during menstruation and she was therefore kept away from possible infection. Through thousands of years and a burgeoning patriarchy, this evolved into a state where women were regarded as 'unclean' during menstruation. They had to observe strict penances, remain in a darkened room and refrain from speaking or laughing loudly. A woman could resume relations with her husband only after a ceremonial bath. Many orthodox households in India still follow this custom of sequestering menstruating women. Ayurveda recommends certain herbs and potions especially for women. Thus liquorice, asafoetida, basil, dried ginger, sesame and hibiscus flowers, among other ingredients, are pounded together to make pastes that regulate the menses. In earlier centuries queens would isolate themselves in palaces built exclusively for this purpose and keep the body healthy with Ayurvedic preparations and a cooling diet.

All ancient civilisations worshipped woman for such inexplicable phenomena as menstruation and procreation. In India she was venerated as *Shakti*, the 'energy that gives power to matter', which is male. Today the power of woman is recognised in the matriarch who rules the family, the wife who controls the household or the career girl who is financially her own mistress.

Even as the ancients glorified womanhood, all women wanted to appear attractive and womanly. They took great pains to find the right plants to massage into their skin and hair, and taught themselves the art of achieving sparkling eyes and graceful feet by borrowing ingredients from the environment. They believed in their own power and stood side by side with men in fields such as mathematics, astronomy and medicine. The *Upanishads*, Hindu texts written between 500 and 900 BC, mention a great mathematician, Gargi, who could put her male counterparts to shame. It was only later that women were subjugated and relegated to the life of second-class citizens. Now it is almost as if we have come full circle. We are once again learning about our own power and are looking to the legacy of our rich past to colour and enrich our lives.

figure

There is no such thing as a perfect figure. Countless charts and magazines have lead us to believe that we must measure up to a table of statistics in order to be considered to have a good figure. Different cultures, too, view body shape and the distribution of fat in different ways. In the West trends have swung between chubby, cherubic figures to the reed-thin bodies of catwalk models. In India a certain amount of female flesh on the bones has always been appreciated – temple architecture and literature, classical to contemporary, stand testimony to that. Sanskrit poets have described their heroine as having a face like a full moon, arms like ivory tusks, a belly that is soft and rounded and thighs like banana

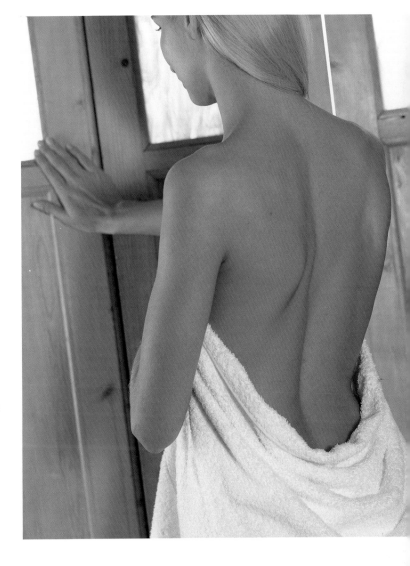

trunks. Large-hipped women are still desired, perhaps because of a primitive instinct that she will be able to produce offspring easily.

Whatever your shape, it is the result of many factors – a reflection of your genetic history as well as your own lifestyle, what and

above

A good figure is in essence, a shape and level of fitness that keeps you happy, healthy and desirable in your own eyes. Learning to love yourself is the first, and most important, step.

how much you eat, whether you exercise, and whether or not you work on your posture. It is true that almost every woman would like to change her shape. Even the near-perfect woman will wish for slimmer thighs or a narrower waist. But when we think of body shape and the ideal weight for ourselves, we first have to understand our body type and accept that certain changes are possible while others are not. The three main types are as follows:

Ectomorph – you have lean, long limbs and are angular with few curves. You do not put on weight easily even if you eat well.

Mesomorph – you have an even figure with no isolated concentration of weight. Your shoulders are broad and muscles well developed.

Endomorph – you are short-limbed, wider-hipped and have more body fat than the other two body types.

It would be ridiculous to state that one type is more desirable than the other just because high fashion requires a particular kind of silhouette for the particular season's collection. Each type has to learn the diet and exercise regimen most suited to her.

posture

The quickest way to lose weight (literally in seconds!), is to straighten your posture. Not only will you look fitter, but you will be healthier too, because your circulation and digestion will receive a boost from the straightening-out of internal systems. In the past, physical activity was a constant presence in daily life everywhere. In Indian villages women still carry loads on the head, which means that the head,

neck back and buttocks are aligned and held upright. The rural woman walks for miles each day in search of food, water and firewood, she balances children on her hip and water pots and wood on her head, she cooks, cleans, dresses, feeds, collects and fetches until nightfall. In comparison her city sister sits hunched at a desk or bends in half while driving a car, turning a knob or pushing a button to start an automated device. All of this means that she does a lot less physical work.

No one teaches us how to sit and stand comfortably and correctly, beyond admonitions in childhood not to slouch. Consider how you are sitting while reading this book – without moving, check the alignment of your body: are your shoulders slumped and your spine curved?

As we grow older, we become set in our postural habits and it gets more and more difficult to correct them. Added to this, we are working against gravity, so straightening up is even more of a burden. Any woman who walks as if she is ten feet tall seems to be saying, 'Look at me,' and she will attract instant attraction and interest, whereas someone who slouches and hangs her head is almost proclaiming that there is nothing of interest about her. – she might as well be invisible. Try walking into a room with your head held high and an easy, upright gait – every head will turn to you and the energy you exude.

standing Divest yourself of all shoulder bags, which temporarily cause an imbalance of weight. Now check your normal standing posture. Most of us adopt a standing stance that does nothing for our allure. We cross our arms in front of our chest (a sure sign that we are wary, self-conscious or defensive) and tend to focus our weight on

one leg, bending the other one at the knee. The shoulders slope down to one side and we keep shifting our weight from one leg to the other in our own fidgety dance. The most impressive way to stand is to:

1 Relax by breathing properly. Yogic exercises begin with good breathing, which means slow, deep, breaths that fill the entire body.

2 Give yourself a good stretch (it is a very good idea to s-t-r-e-t-c-h the body completely on waking: it seems to set the pace for a fitter day).

3 Stand with your feet a few inches apart and really 'ground' your toes. This will be difficult in shoes, so practise barefoot at first. It is impossible to achieve perfect balance

when your feet are close together – and it looks appropriate only if you are in uniform.

4 Slowly push your shoulders back without shifting your ribs or back, till your shoulders are in line with your neck.

5 If you are used to standing with your bottom slightly pushed out, pull it in till it feels as if it is line with your heels.

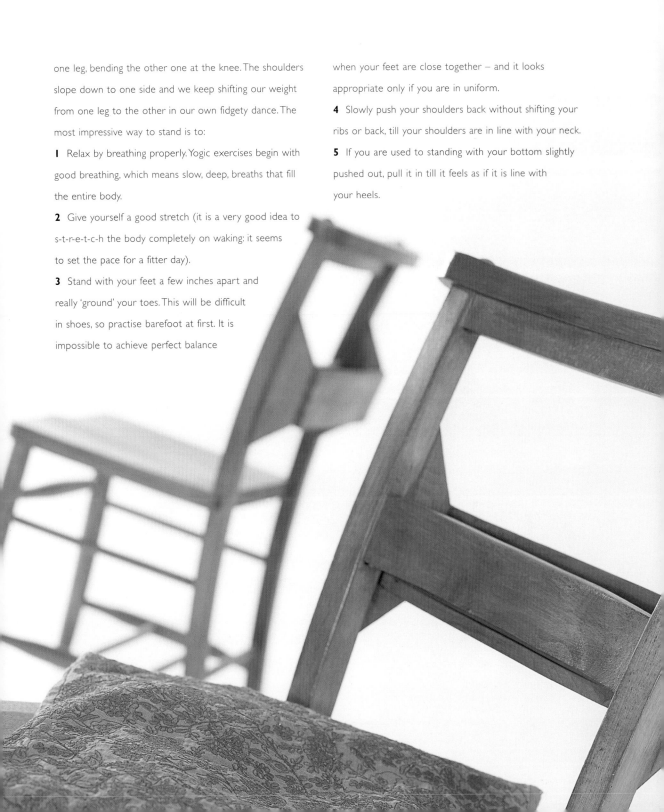

6 Raise your chin to make your neck long and elegant and give yourself an air of confidence.

walking

It is not at all easy to relearn how to walk in adulthood. A little daily practice, however, will reap dividends. Try the following as you walk into a busy room:

1 Lead with your hips and not your tummy, shoulders or head. Tighten your bottom and move ahead in long, graceful strides.

2 Walk slowly and take measured steps. Have you ever watched a tigress move? She walks at a leisurely pace but with supreme grace, giving an observer enough time to admire and enjoy her amazing beauty.

3 Keep your arms close to your sides. There is no need to swish them or flap them about. A small movement of straightened arms is all that is required to propel you.

4 When entering a crowded room, raise your chin and pause for a deep breath at the entrance. It also helps to swing your eyes around and survey the proceedings before stepping into the room. To make a real impact, you must give everyone enough time to notice you; it really is that simple. In India, there are several classical dance styles, one of which is *Mohini-attam*, the dance of the enchantress. As part of this very sensuous dance, the dancer walks in a series of decorative steps that involve a slight swaying of the hips, swinging of the arms, turning of the neck and shooting tempting glances with heavy-lidded eyes – all very seductive indeed!

Young students of dance are taught how to walk with exaggerated style so that they almost resemble gliding swans or strutting peacocks.

sitting

We have all been taught 'to cross our legs and sit like a lady', but have you ever thought what prolonged periods of such sitting do to the posture or, more importantly, to the circulation? There is a graceful way of sitting without crunching up the body:

1 Walk to the front of a chair and turn around so that your back is to it.

2 Feeling the front of the chair with the back of your legs, lower yourself with a straight back and with your tummy muscles held in. Do not fold into a chair, collapse into it or use your hands to manoeuvre the movement.

3 Now position your feet a few inches apart with the knees straight in front. Tilt your pelvis ever so slightly to the front. This will automatically lengthen the lower spine and ease any tension that has built up there.

4 Imagine the head being pulled towards the sky very gently. This should elongate your neck, your stomach muscles should tighten and the ribcage should lift, making deep breathing easier. All this helps to 'open out' the digestive system. An efficient digestion is reflected positively in the skin, hair and eyes.

The traditional Indian style of seating is the *baithak*, which comprises a mat or mattress on the floor with a scattering of cushions. Before colonisation this was where all Indians sat to work, rest or eat. The cross-legged, yogic 'lotus position' has become a symbol of tranquillity and health, as it allows all the body functions and energies to harmonise. In India practitioners of the traditional arts, such as music or dance, still sit on the floor, their backs and shoulders held up and their hips tucked under in a pose of perfect alignment and comfort.

eating sensibly

According to the *Charak Samhita*, one of the oldest Sanskrit texts on Ayurveda written approximately between AD 90 and 180, 'Our body is a result of food, so also disease is caused by food. Right food causes *sukha* (health) and wrong food causes *dukha* (disease).' In India we are brought up with the Ayurvedic knowledge of what foods to eat for optimum health, what food combinations may lead to ill-health, how to aid digestion with herbs and how to change the diet incorporating seasonal fruits and vegetables to counter the extremes of weather. The reverence we have for nature – its herbs, fruits and flowers – is neither super-stitious nor a mere appreciation of beauty. Above all, it is an innate understanding of the power of plants and how we can fine-tune our mind and body with their natural energy.

During my childhood, in the first few days of winter, when early mists would begin to swirl in from the Arabian Sea into Bombay, my grandmother would start making 'winter specials' – sesame and jaggery crackle, ginger fudge and garlic pickle, all foods that are known to produce heat in the body.

An important concept of ayurveda is the *ushman* or 'temperature inherent in all foods. All foods are classified as *ushna* (hot) or *sheeta* (cold) and the two words are used liberally whenever Indians converse about food. Balancing the amount of hot and cold foods leads to good health and beauty. Heat is the property of fire and air. It warms, melts, disperses and evaporates and is said to be created by 'hot' foods, anger, worry, tension or hyper-activity. People with 'heaty' dispositions are easily tired, always thirsty, hate the summer and are constantly agitated. They need, 'cooling', foods such as lemons, oranges (contrary to what seems

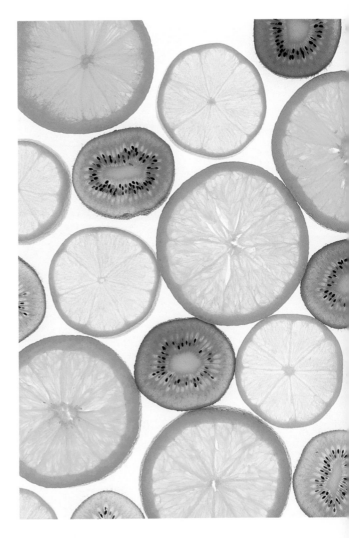

obvious, citrus fruits, however acidic, are cooling), pears, strawberries, cucumber, beetroot, tomatoes, lettuce, rice, oatmeal, coffee, beer, beef, veal, fish, milk, yoghurt, cheese and buttermilk. On the other hand, 'cold' is a property of earth and water. It freezes, extinguishes or contracts and is created by 'cold' foods, too much relaxation or too much exercise. People who have a 'cold' temperament have a

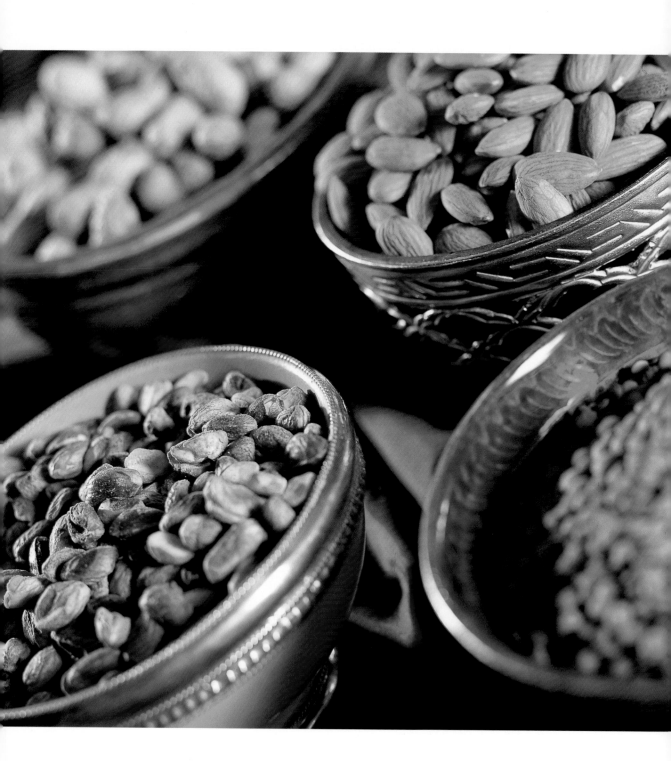

weak digestion, catarrh and a tendency to influenza and pneumonia. They should eat 'hot' foods such as apples, figs, dates (very good), cabbage, cauliflower, onions, garlic, carrots, potatoes, wheat products, pasta, tea, cocoa, whisky, lamb, chicken, pork, butter, cream, eggs, honey and olive oil. Balancing these different foods helps to regulate the various processes of the body.

Ayurveda has certain rules regarding eating. One must chew slowly and carefully while thinking pleasant thoughts. This helps digestion and generates a sense of well-being. Fluids drunk before a meal delay digestion and cause leanness, those drunk during the meal promote digestion and those drunk after a meal cause obesity. One must be surrounded by pleasant things while eating as tastes are linked to emotion. What emotion is to the mind, taste is to the body. This is evident in the Sanskrit word *rasa*, which means taste as well as emotion. A conducive environment is as important as what you do after eating. 'After meals, sitting causes laziness, lying adds to body weight, walking slowly increases life (health), but if you run immediately after meals, your death also runs after you,' advises an ancient Sanskrit saying. On a day-to-day basis, we are advised to regulate the various ingredients of our diet.

protein On average adults, with the exception of
pregnant women, do not need as much protein as children or teenagers. The body requires protein for growth as well as for repairing tissues, and this is assimilated in the form of twenty-two vital amino acids. Of these, eight cannot be made by the body and must be absorbed from the food we eat, food such as eggs, fish, meat, pulses and nuts. For vegetarians getting sufficient protein is an important consideration. In the West vegetarianism still has a slightly 'faddy' image, though things are changing.

In India, however, where 85 percent of the population are Hindus, many of whom for religious reasons choose not to eat meat, vegetarianism is simply not an issue – a certain section of society is vegetarian, the other is not. The Indian diet is beautifully equipped to provide all the protein required nutritionally for health and well-being. Studies have shown that soya has more protein, weight for weight, than some meats. Lentils, milk products and nuts are the protein-rich components of an Indian meal. A typical vegetarian meal might consist of a bowl of *dal* (lentils), a bowl of yoghurt and a nutty dessert such as almond *kulfi* (ice-cream) to accompany the 'starchy' and 'fatty' elements, so as to make up a balanced, wholesome and tasty meal. Another plus point is that vegetarians have lower cholesterol levels and are healthier and slimmer than their meat-eating sisters, thus exploding a myth that has thrived in the West, which claims that a meal is not a meal without meat.

carbohydrates Contemporary aesthetics
demand that grains be milled and 'purified' to look and taste better. This is a real shame as the processes involve stripping away the oils and bran, both of which are extremely nutritious. In India the staple foods are rice and wheat. Wheat is ground whole into flour and then used

left

Nuts such as lime green pistachios, peanuts and honey-coloured almonds provide essential protein in a vegetarian diet. Lentils too are a rich source of protein.

for making various breads such as *poories* and *rotis*. Rice too is left unpolished to retain its goodness. Refined flour is used sparingly and in most cases it is perfectly acceptable to substitute it with wholewheat flour.

fats Every ayurvedic text on diet extols the benefits of fat in that it provides energy, boosts brain function and is essential for healthy bones and tissues. While we all need some fat, however, we certainly do not need the amounts that most of us consume today. In fact, in most parts of the world, food becomes richer in direct proportion to the fat used in its cooking. Here are some simple tips to reduce your fat intake:

• Cut down on red meat and choose lean, white meat such as chicken or fish. Grill rather than fry, bake with little or no fat rather than roast. Experiment with fat-free sauces or go without them completely.

• Watch your egg intake. An egg a day is fine if your cholesterol levels are fine, otherwise stick to no more than three eggs a week.

• Drink skimmed milk instead of full-cream milk. You do not need cream at all (no, not even with strawberries – use it on your face instead!).

• Watch the amount of butter you put on your bread, the oil you use in cooking and the fat content of offals such as liver, kidney and heart.

my own diet for health & beauty

There are certain times in life when each of us feels fat, dingy and dull. All our systems need a perk and we like this to happen in a short time without any health hazards. For such times in my own life I have devised a diet based on Ayurveda and the wisdom of my ancestors as well as personal experience. I cannot stand diets which tell me how much of what to eat at each meal. I find them stifling and impractical, and I give up by the second or third day. What I do is this. For one month I:

• Cut out all refined flour, which means no white bread, cakes, sauces or pancakes.

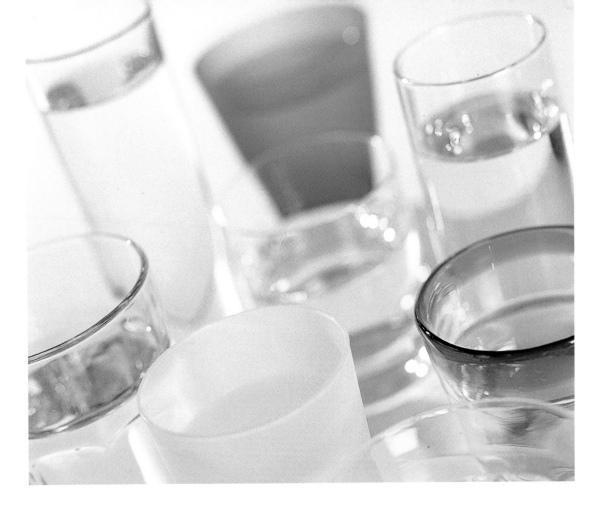

• Cut out all refined sugar. I love it but I do not need it and it will only add weight, ruin my teeth and make me prone to diabetes or even heart disease. I fulfil the persistent demands of my sweet tooth with delicious alternatives such as fruit, fresh juices, jaggery or molasses. Jaggery is dehydrated sugar cane juice, which is not refined. It retains all the qualities of the juice itself and has a caramel-like musky aroma. It is widely available in Indian shops all over the world.

• Cut out most fat – butter, ghee, cheese and oil. I do eat chicken and fish, so that their natural oils lubricate the system. My theory is that the body should start to use up reserves of fat stored within it so that I lose weight.

• Apart from all this, I drink plenty of water or *lassi* (made by mixing a spoonful of yoghurt in a glass of water) and no wine, beer or spirits. I also cut down on salt (we need only about a gram a day) by eliminating processed foods and by adding a minimum amount to my cooking. A multi-vitamin plus iron pill a day boosts my energy through the day.

Although all this may sound quite harsh, you will find that within a few days, that your body will adjust to your new diet and any hunger pangs will reduce. At the end of the month, I guarantee you will feel healthier, your skin and eyes will radiate with a sense of well-being and the compliments will come in thick and fast! However, as any dietitian will recommend, always consult your own doctor before you embark on this diet – especially if you have or have in the past had any medical problems, or if you are in any doubt whatsoever.

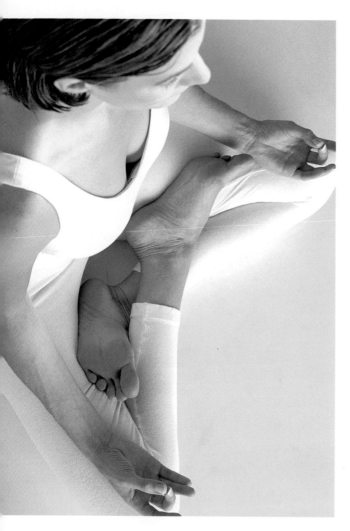

exercise

I trained in *Bharata Natyam*, a style of Indian classical dance, for more than twenty-two years. During this time my body was honed and taught to move gracefully. I was also taught the value of good breathing and how it could increase my stamina and boost my energy levels. My 'guru' would patiently explain to me, as I sat massaging my weary feet

each evening, that in order to dance effortlessly for two hours on stage it was necessary for me to practise each day for at least eight hours – two hours would then seem like child's play!

Energy generates more energy. There is no beauty routine more rewarding than an exercise or fitness programme, as this reflects on our ability to handle stress, limbers up while firming the body, increases resistance to disease and makes us feel vibrant and youthful. The fitter you are, the more active you will be. If you are feeling lethargic, try putting on a tape and dancing for fifteen minutes – you will emerge refreshed and ready to go.

Contrary to what many of us believe, especially when we are unfit, all exercise need not be boring. You may find swimming exhilarating, others may feel that a jog in the fresh air is as close as they will get to flying free. Even brisk walking is beneficial – and burns 300–350 calories an hour. Whatever you choose, exercise is a must, for beauty begins within and shows results on the outside.

That exercise is essential to life is evident in the ancient physical and mental discipline of yoga. It is believed that the word 'yoga' derives from the root *yuj*, which means to join, symbolising the union of the human soul with the Universal One. Yoga is not simply a method of exercise; there are several forms of yoga that can be practised depending on what is to be attained. *Jnana-yoga* is salvation through knowledge, *karma-yoga* is liberation through work and *mantra-yoga* is contemplation on the sound and vibrations of chanting. One of the most popular forms is *hatha-yoga*, which involves a physical culture. The symbol *ha* represents the sun and *tha* the moon and these together represent the polarity in each individual, the two genders present in each of us, two breaths in two nostrils and so on. *Hatha-yoga* has within its repertoire hundreds of body positions, for even the eyes and the tongue, that harmonise the functions of the body and alleviate stress and disease.

Yoga is gentle enough to suit people of all ages and at any level of fitness, although it is advisable to seek your doctor's advice before you start. Some people think that because yoga is slow-paced, it is passive and will not show results for a very long time. However, the technique requires the building-up of holding power and stamina, both of which have deep-reaching effects. We have all heard of Indian yogis who levitate, walk on burning coals, or alter their pulse rate at will. This is not to say that all of us should aspire to these feats of discipline and dedication, but there is hardly any doubt that with the regular practice of yoga the body and the mind can be elevated to great levels of power and accomplishment.

Yoga helps mainly by stretching the muscles, which can become cramped with age or lack of use. One of India's best-known yogis, Dhirendra Bramhachari, who was the personal instructor of Mrs Indira Gandhi, the first Indian woman prime minister, was a fit, youthful man even in his seventies. As part of my dance training I learnt a warm-up routine that is based on yoga. This really loosened my muscles and got me ready for the session. Here is how I began:

surya namaskar (saluting the sun)

1 Stand with your feet together and arms at your side. Push the shoulders back and tuck in your pelvis. Feel the ground with your bare feet.

2 Join the hands, palm to palm, in front of your chest and inhale deeply. Hold for a minute and breathe out.

3 Swing the arms over the head, breathe out and bend forward to place the palms flat on the floor. If this is difficult, go as far as you can, but if the floor is easily reachable, stretch your forehead to your knees.

4 In one fluid movement, bend the right knee and stretch your left leg straight behind while placing your palms flat on the floor, on either side of your right foot. Arch your back and lift your chin to the ceiling.

5 Lower the chin and extend your right leg to join the left, keeping the body tense and the knees off the ground.

6 Dip your head between your arms in an arc and straighten the torso to look straight ahead of you. Alternate your breathing with each move – in, out, in, out.

7 Your pelvis, knees and toes should be flat on the ground, arms stretched taut and breathing even.

8 Breathe out and lift yourself to a position where the feet are wide apart on the ground, the bottom is raised to the sky and the head is dropped between the arms as the palms take the support of the floor.

9 Start working back, one step at a time, quite slowly, till you regain your original standing position.

As part of the warm-up, we continued with *halasana* (the plough) and *sarvangasana* (shoulder stand), ending with *shavasana* (the corpse). Yogic *asanas* or poses have to be practised until you can do them correctly. Never go into the difficult ones without giving your body time to warm up. The lotus pose (see picture far left) helps to focus one's energy and mind to set the mood for the day ahead.

Choose a form of exercise that you enjoy so you will be motivated to keep on doing it. It should be something that is safe and that will help you to work yourself to an optimum individual shape within a time frame you set for yourself.

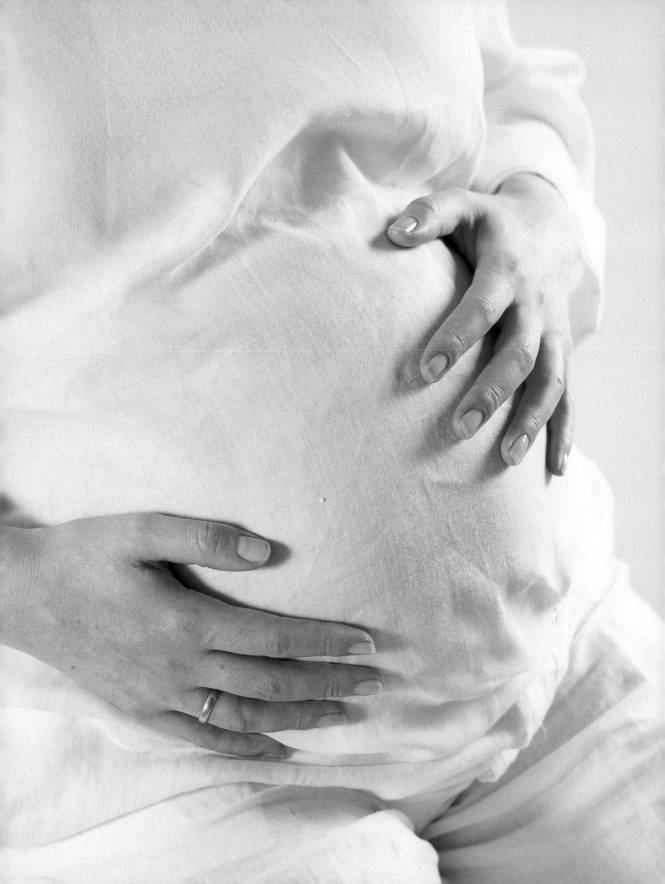

'Being happy in mind, here mount the bed; give birth to children for me, your husband' *Atharvaveda – Hindu text written c. 900–500 BC*

pregnancy

Every ancient civilisation of the world has worshipped women in the form of a Mother Goddess. In India, she was Shakti, the energy and power that fuelled every living being. Around 2300 BC in Sumeria, now Iraq, she was Queen of Heaven and priests composed hymns that revered her 'lap of honey' and 'the natural bounty that poured forth from her womb'. Rosalind Miles writes in The Women's History of the World, 'But the real key lies where the exaggerated breasts and belly of the earliest images of women direct us to look, in the miracle of birth.' A woman's ability to procreate was considered magical and odes were composed about her fertility and benevolence.

In the *Padmapuran*, an ancient Hindu text, the pregnant woman merited special care as she was the 'vessel' for the baby, 'She should not bathe in a river, nor be mentally disturbed… she should not be always sleeping or dormant…' From the time of the Vedas, motherhood was put on the highest pedestal and every mother-to-be was treated like a princess.

In the hustle and bustle of modern life all Indians still celebrate certain days with ceremonies and rituals. Some of these specifically revolve around women and their need to be glamorous and beautiful. One of the most important rituals in a Hindu woman's life is the *Seemant*, which is celebrated in the seventh month of her pregnancy. The mother-to-be is dressed in jewel-coloured silks and dazzling gold jewellery to resemble a bride. Part of the purpose of this ritual, mentioned in texts dating between 900 and 500 BC, was to make the pregnant woman feel beautiful during a time when she might feel large or ungainly. Thus, during the ceremony, the husband addresses his wife as 'O, of beautiful colour', or as 'Supesha', which means 'of beautiful limbs'. The ceremony itself is celebrated with feasts of foods that are green in colour. In fact the day is dominated by the colour green, which represents fertility in nature. The mother-to-be wears green glass bangles and serves food such as spinach fritters, coriander squares and sweet pistachio and milk fudge to her friends. Older married women present her with flowers and a coconut, a symbol of good luck and plenty.

Indian mythology is full of stories that centre around the fertility of women. Owing to the awesome ability to reproduce, women could become pregnant by 'invoking the blessings of the gods' (*Mahabharata*), eating blessed food (*Ramayana*), or even by severe penances.

The concept of motherhood is celebrated in every aspect of Indian life. A mother is respected and has considerable control over the physical and emotional destiny of her children. She is seen as strong, forgiving, nurturing, protective and beautiful and therefore epithets such as Mother Earth (for her fruitfulness), Mother India (for her power and grace) and Mother Nature (for her ability to procreate) abound in everyday conversation. In the long, chequered history of India, mothers have played an important part. In the epic *Mahabharata* it was Kunti, the mother of the five heroes, the Pandavas; in the middle of the seventeenth century it was Jijamata, the mother of the Maratha ruler Shivaji; and in the nineteenth century, the Begum of Bhopal. Even today most Indians will seek the blessings and approval of their parents, most particularly of their mother, before embarking on a new project.

Exalted status apart, any woman who has ever been pregnant will know that it is a time of ups and downs, when you may feel very sick but can radiate with a glow that sings out health and vitality. Overall it is generally accepted that women become more beautiful during pregnancy. The extra hormones pouring into the bloodstream enhance femininity and make women look serene and sparkling. In fact, how wonderful it would be if we could have the positive side effects of pregnancy throughout our lives!

There are some who are lucky and literally sail through the nine months, but others are not so fortunate – their skin breaks out in spots, their hair becomes difficult and tiredness discourages them. But a positive, excited outlook is essential in pregnancy. This is a very special time in your life – one that may not repeat itself often and it is up to you to feel calm, centred and really beautiful inside out.

eating

The well-being of her baby is every mother's prime concern. To give your baby the best possible start in life, make yourself fit and healthy before you conceive. Thousands of years ago, when life was lived according to a set of rules as written in the sacred books, the Hindus followed a ritual called *Garbhadhana* or conception. Prior to this the woman was fed fortifying herbs such as liquorice and the root of *shatavari* (wild asparagus) to strengthen her. (In fact *shatavari* is prescribed by Ayurveda to increase fertility. It is still given to nursing mothers as it increases the quantity and quality of breast milk.) There were also ceremonies at which the woman would be massaged with oils that would tone her muscles and make her strong enough to nurture a foetus.

It is just as important to prepare yourself well for pregnancy today. Good muscle tone and healthy internal systems will ensure that childbirth itself will be easier and recovery quicker. Putting on weight is a natural result of pregnancy, but doctors recommend that no more than 9kg (20lb) should be gained so that getting back into shape is easier. If you are thinking of becoming pregnant, this is a good time to get to your ideal weight. Being too thin will mean that you may not be able to provide adequate nourishment for the baby and excess weight at this stage makes you prone to putting on more during the pregnancy. Dieting is, however, absolutely taboo as are erratic eating habits, so get fit with a super exercise regiment and a healthy, nutritious diet.

Smoking or drinking is never beneficial to the developing baby, so this is a good time to review your habits. A baby's heart rate can increase by 30 percent during cigarette smoking by the mother.

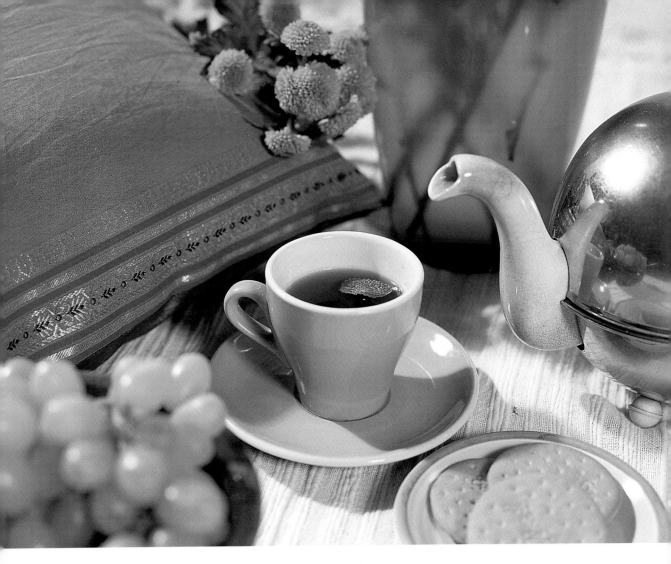

It is believed that if a pregnant woman looks at beautiful things, her baby will be beautiful too. In India female relatives will decorate a pregnant woman's room with pictures of baby Krishna, as well as pictures of other gods and goddesses.

Along with the mind, the body is kept calm with good food. Mint tea, made by simply adding a sprig of fresh mint to Indian tea, is given to overcome morning sickness. Doctors also recommend a plain biscuit with tea before getting out of bed. Eat small, bland meals frequently through the day to cope with nausea.

skin

Pregnancy is a time of change for the skin – it will stretch in places and grow in others, and you will need to take extra care that it remains in good condition. Your skin may improve beyond belief, especially if it was spotty or blemished to begin with, but around the fourth month you are likely to develop fine, pink lines called stretch marks on your abdomen, buttocks, thighs and arms. These happen deep under the skin in the dermal layer, so massaging creams into the skin will only help to minimise their appearance. The ability of the skin to withstand the

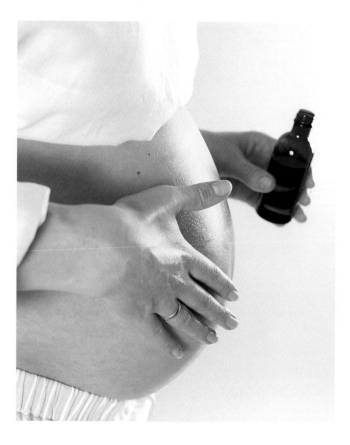

and collagen that are both responsible for the skin's tenacity and elasticity. Although stretch marks are permanent, they will fade from pink to a translucent, silvery colour that may blend into your skin tone.

During this time especially, your skin is also going to reveal whether you live on a diet of junk food or health treats, so watch what you eat. Vitamin A is vital for the skin's satiny texture. One good-sized carrot a day should fulfil your daily requirement, but do consult your doctor for more individual dietary needs. Vitamin A is plentiful in dark green or golden vegetables, so try spinach, carrots and pumpkin. I also found that crunching a carrot helped me keep my extreme sickness at bay, at least temporarily. A famine of vitamin B6, found abundantly in pork and bananas, gives you oily, spotty skin, and a shortage of niacin will make the skin dry. Niacin-rich foods are chicken, liver and mushrooms. Foods rich in vitamin C help the skin look fresh and smooth, as I have found from personal experience. Nearly all vegetables contain some vitamin C, but especially good sources are citrus fruits (oranges are excellent), leafy, green vegetables, strawberries and papayas. Vitamin E is known as the 'skin vitamin' because it delays ageing and aids the circulation of blood: this helps in the renewal of skin to keep it radiant. Eat soya foods, wheatgerm and wheatgerm oil for your daily requirement of vitamin E.

above
A daily massage with almond oil from early pregnancy will help to arrest the onset of stretch marks.

right
A basket of ripe, juicy mangoes bursting with the goodness of vitamin A and C offer tempting promises of sunshine and health.

tension of stretching is genetically influenced and there is only very little you can do to try to change this: if your grandmother and mother developed stretch marks, in all likelihood you will too. However, regular massage with almond oil will lubricate the skin and make it more supple and able to cope with the unbelievable amount of stretching that it will have to go through. You can also eat foods rich in zinc, such as seafood, which, together with vitamins B6 and C, participates in the production of elastin

hair

A boost in the growth of your hair is a natural and wonderful bonus during pregnancy. Your hair flourishes when you eat a diet rich in protein, vitamin B, iron and iodine. Protein is easily available in lean meat, poultry, eggs, fish, nuts (check with your doctor about eating nuts during pregnancy, though: some are a precursor to allergy) and beans. Brewer's yeast is one of the best sources of vitamin B – you can take up to six tablets daily when not pregnant, but check with your doctor for your specific requirement during pregnancy. Make up your iron requirement with grills or stews of red meat, lentils and dried fruit. Eat foods rich in vitamin C with your meal as this will make absorption of iron by the body four times more efficient. This is probably why Indians squeeze lemon juice over their grilled kebabs and tandoori chicken! Tannin has the reverse effect, so avoid tea, which is full of it. Iodine boosts circulation in the scalp and can be found in plenty in seafood. In fact a scalp massage of iodine and castor oil on alternate days for four days will stop hair fall.

constipation

The most common causes of constipation are an unbalanced diet and a lack of exercise and fresh air. Anyone who has been constipated knows the feeling of heaviness and lethargy, headaches, heartburn and bad breath that accompany it. In pregnancy, hormone changes can encourage constipation. Straining when constipated is never a good idea, and straining during pregnancy increases the chances of developing haemorrhoids, which also sometimes occur after the heavy straining of childbirth.

The easiest way to help yourself is to start incorporating fibre-rich foods such as fruit (pears and apples work wonders), vegetables and bran (in cereals and breads) into your diet. Even while not pregnant, many women I know swear by a banana a day and I have given fresh, purple figs to my little children with wonderfully immediate results! My grandmother's remedy was a handful of fat, shiny raisins that she would stuff into my tiny palm. I loved the treat, never realising that it was 'medicine'.

Another pleasant food that finds a high place in Ayurveda is yoghurt. Indian meals end with yoghurt (yoghurt and

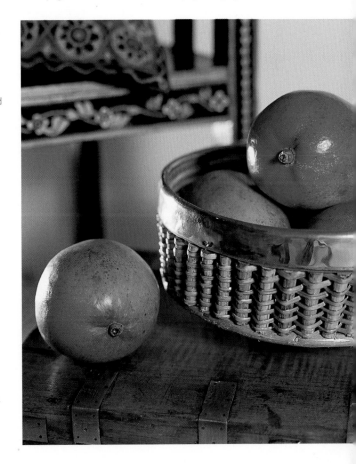

Feeling her baby's movements is a special moment between mother and child. A mother's sense of well-being will contribute to a safe and enjoyable pregnancy, which is a time when most women feel content and peaceful.

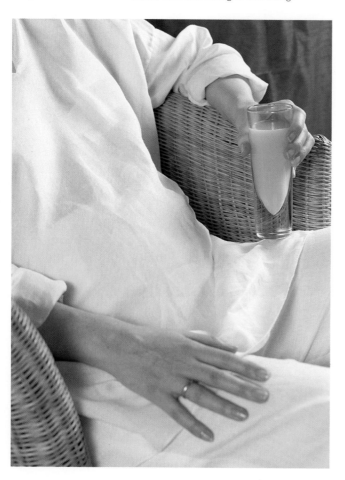

rice in south India; a glass of *lassi* or creamy buttermilk in the north), which is considered one of the best digestives because of all the enzymes and lactic ferments it contains. A couple of tablespoons of live (bio) yoghurt stirred into a glass of water is a natural and gentle laxative. It is also important to get yourself into the habit of opening your bowels regularly. It will tell instantly in your skin, fitness, smile and feeling of well-being.

weight gain

Pregnancy is traditionally a time when a woman looks her best in spite of a marked gain in weight. In Indian mythology the goddess Aditi, mother of all the major gods and the sustainer of all existence, is so large in her manifestation of pregnancy and childbearing that she is personified as the limitless expanse of the universe. From her vast belly are said to arise the *adityas* or celestial deities who represent the twelve signs of the Indian zodiac.

Most women gain hardly any weight in the first three months. From the fourth month, as the foetus begins its rapid growth, the mother too begins to put on weight. This comes from a growing placenta and increasing amniotic fluid, the supplementing of the breast tissue and the laying down of reserves of fat for the latter part of the pregnancy.

Around the third trimester, or seventh month, a woman may carry up to 6–7kg (13–15lb) more than her usual weight, and as the date of confinement draws nearer the volume of blood circulating in the body rises one and a half times. Needless to say, by the end of the term, all women feel lethargic and breathless, lose their balance easily and find it difficult to do up their shoes or give themselves a pedicure.

Doctors recommend that it should take about nine months after childbirth for a woman to come back to shape, six if she is basically fit and supple. Some of the additional weight will be seen in deposits around the breast tissue. The resulting extra cleavage is usually welcome, but supporting the weight of newly increased breasts is essential if you want to prevent them drooping later in life. Buy a well fitting bra early in pregnancy and perhaps a light, stretchy one to wear at night if their weight makes you uncomfortable. However much you are tempted to do away with your bra (many women feel that the elastic is too restrictive on a growing chest), never give in. A supportive bra at this time is vital in helping to keep the shape and tone of the breasts.

Stretch marks (see pages 119–20) rise with the increase in weight, so it makes sense to watch your weight during pregnancy. Some women find that weight loss after pregnancy begins in earnest only when breastfeeding ends. However, we were always told by the matriarchs in our family that breastfeeding 'melted away the fat' and that one should breastfeed for as long as possible. The theory behind this is that body stores of fats and carbohydrates are used in the production of breast milk. Moreover, as the baby suckles, the mother produces hormones which help the uterus to contract and therefore the tummy to become flat faster. The myth that breastfeeding causes the breasts to droop or sag has created enough confusion in the minds of young mothers. The fact is that changes in the shape or size of the breast are a result of pregnancy and not of breast-feeding, so it makes good sense to wear a well-fitting bra throughout. According to Ayurveda, the herbs *shatavari* (*Asparagus racemosus* or wild asparagus) is like ambrosia for a new mother. It tones up the breast muscles significantly while increasing the quantity and quality of milk. Several Sanskrit texts describe the herb as *stanyakari* or 'breast enhancing' and it is also known to increase fertility.

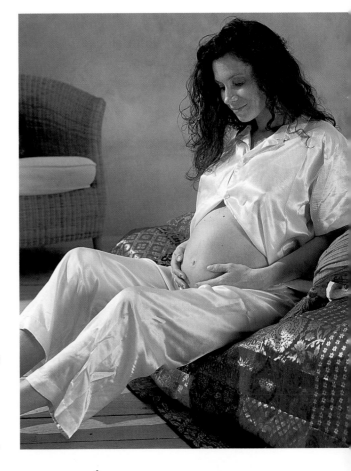

exercise

Pregnancy brings on innumerable and unexpected changes in every woman's body. Fitness at this time is of utmost importance, not only to keep a check on unnecessary increase in weight, but also to ensure that the muscles are supple and strong for easy childbirth. I cannot begin to explain how much smoother my own two deliveries were because of years of dance training and practice. The abdomen, lower back and breathing, all of which come into play during intensive rehearsal and performance, stood by me wonderfully in the delivery room. Getting back to shape was that much simpler as well – more so with my firstborn; I actually took him on tour when he was just four months old!

If you do not normally participate in sports or physical activity, pregnancy is a good time to start. Of course, you must consult your own doctor at every stage. In the old Sanskrit scriptures such as the *Padmapurana* (composed *c.* AD 1100) or the *Garbhopanishad* (a series of discourses on embryology, composed *c.* 400–200 BC), pregnant women were advised against 'sitting on a pestle or mace, bathing in a river, mounting a horse or elephant, mountain climbing, swift walking, journeying in a bullock-cart, sitting like a cock…' These precautions were even prescribed by Ayurvedic physicians such as Sushruta (AD 350) to ensure

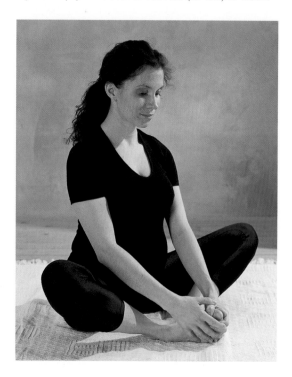

complete safety and health of the mother-to-be. However, we now live in an age when the benefits of fitness have been sufficiently proved and proper exercise during pregnancy may help to alleviate some of the discomfort and minor ailments that come along during this time. For some women staying in shape during pregnancy is doubly difficult; perhaps it is because they follow misguided advice and 'eat for two'! This will only make *you* increase in size, not your baby.

Here are some gentle exercises to build up into a routine. Be careful not to overdo any of them, never strain, listen to your body and always consult your practitioner first.

Exercise A (LEFT)

1 Sit upright on the floor and join the soles of your feet, keeping your knees apart.

2 Hold your toes together and slowly rotate your neck forwards, left, back, right and forwards. Do this three times clockwise, then thee times anti-clockwise.

3 Make small back-to-front arcs with the shoulders then repeat front to back. Do not forget to breathe while exercising.

Exercise B

1 Stretch your legs out in front of you. Support yourself by placing your palms flat on the floor beside your hips. Point your toes, then flex them.

2 Spread your legs apart slowly. Draw small circles in the air with your toes, exercising your ankles and feet.

3 Breathe in and reach over with both hands towards the right foot, breathing out as you bend. Go only as far as is comfortable. Repeat this towards the left foot.

4 Hold both feet, tighten the legs and feel the stretch in the legs, back and arms.

Exercise C

I Sit up straight with your legs wide apart. Hold your arms out at shoulder height and swing them in, bringing the hands to the shoulders in an upward arc.

2 Swing your arms down and around to the back and fold them across your back, thus stretching the shoulder and back muscles.

Exercise D

I Cross your legs, breathe in and lift your arms to the ceiling, breathing out slowly as you do so. Stretch.

2 Keep the arms stretched up, then gently lean over to the right, breathing in as you go and out as you come to your upright position. Repeat on the left.

Exercise E (TOP RIGHT)

I Kneel on the floor on all fours. Breathe in, lift the left leg and slowly stretch it out behind you while you breathe out. Repeat for the right leg.

2 Arch the back cat-fashion, first towards the floor then up towards the ceiling.

3 Drop down to the floor and bring in your chin to your knees like a tortoise withdrawn into its shell. Breathe in to a count of five and out to another count of five.

Exercise F

I Stand with your feet apart, breathe in and lift your arms over your head. Breathe out and bend forwards as far as you can go.

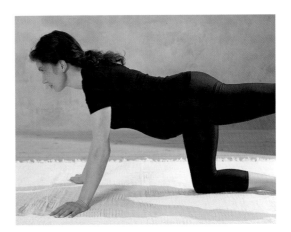

2 Bend your knees and rest your palms on the floor. Try to use your lower back muscles and not your palms to help you come to an upright position. This means that you should straighten up from the waist and not the shoulders.

Exercise G

I Stand with your feet hip distance apart, toes turned slightly outwards. Slowly breathe in, lift your arms to shoulder height and lower yourself a bit as you bend your knees. Hold this position as you exhale to a count of five.

2 Keep standing with your feet apart. Breathe in and reach for your left foot with your left hand, exhaling as you go. Repeat on the right foot.

Exercise H

Relax by lying down on your side and raising one knee onto a pillow. This takes the pressure off the abdomen and uterus and allows blood to circulate more freely. Breathe slowly and deeply.

breathing

The earliest practitioners of yoga, including Patanjali (c. 200 BC), believed in the wonderful results of breath control or *pranayama*. Proper breathing, they said, cleansed and purified the internal vessels and vitalised the energy centres of the body. Controlled breathing, according to the treatise *Yoga-sutra*, written by Patanjali, has the power to make the face 'glow like the sun'.

Breathing supplies oxygen that is vital to life, to every tiny cell of the body. Just because it seems to happen automatically does not mean that you are breathing in the best possible manner or that you cannot improve your technique. Inadequate breathers are often lethargic, anxious or even prone to frequent headaches. They take in only short breaths that skim off the top of the lungs, leaving a large volume of carbon dioxide.

If you are breathing properly, your tummy and ribcage should expand on inhalation and deflate on exhalation. In the yogic stance of *shavasana* or 'the corpse', attention is focused on the breathing as you lie on your back on the floor in a relaxed pose. Here the aim is to release all tension from the mind as well as the body and concentrate on the flow of air into the body and out. A steady rhythm is established and the senses become calm but still remain very sharp.

Accomplished yogis actually use *pranayama* in order to regulate their body processes –

breath control helps them to slow down the heart rate or to lower the blood pressure. Patanjali mentions in his *Yoga-sutra* that 'the central vital breath rises through the middle channel, first like an ant, slowly; then like a frog leaping and finally like a bird flying upwards, and enters the centre of the thousand petals at the top of the head. When this is achieved, life may be prolonged indefinitely…'

Breathing properly during pregnancy needs careful practice. As the foetus grows and the tummy seems to push into the chest, breathing becomes short and laboured. Practise your breathing each day: sit in a comfortable upright position and breathe in slowly but deeply. Hold for a count of three. Exhale and hold for a count of three. Do this at least ten times, bearing in mind that this exercise should be comfortable and never strenuous. Apart from feeling relaxed, you will reap the rich rewards of this routine during labour.

make the most of yourself

In India the 'bloom' on a young married woman's face is always at the centre of gentle teasing and probing about possible 'good news'. An air of happiness and excitement surrounds the expectant mother. She is made a great fuss of and all her female relatives come together to

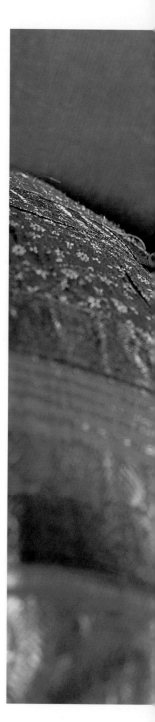

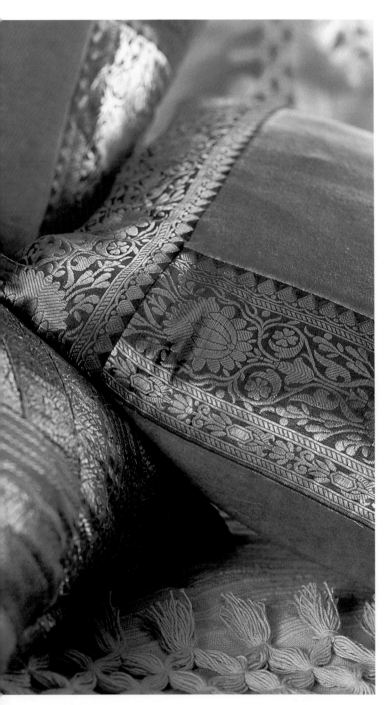

look after her. Her mother-in-law organises a 'massage-wali', a woman who comes every day to rub smooth, rich herbal creams and oils into her skin and gently knead away the aches from her lower back and feet. The expectant mother's aunts send her gifts of soothing music and pleasant story-books, while her mother makes her a box of her favourite food or a special titbit nearly every day. A pregnant woman's cravings are taken very seriously indeed – not fulfilling these, it is believed, will make the baby dissatisfied and cranky. The mother's every request is received with great enthusiasm and her relatives vie with each other to conjure up her latest culinary wish. Her husband brings home little baskets of fresh fruit – figs, grapes, oranges, guavas or mangoes. Papayas and pineapples are strictly taboo as they produce too much heat in the body and are said to cause a woman to miscarry. The first food on my wish list during pregnancies was pineapple, only because I was not allowed it!

All her relatives and friends invite the expectant mother to elaborate lunches and dinners and it is a real effort for her to keep in shape. She is decorated with garlands of fresh flowers and dressed in silks and jewels. Her family regularly takes her to a temple to focus her energies, to open-air music concerts under the stars to relax her mind and to funny Hindi films for a giggle. She is spoilt silly and does not need to lift a finger during the nine months.

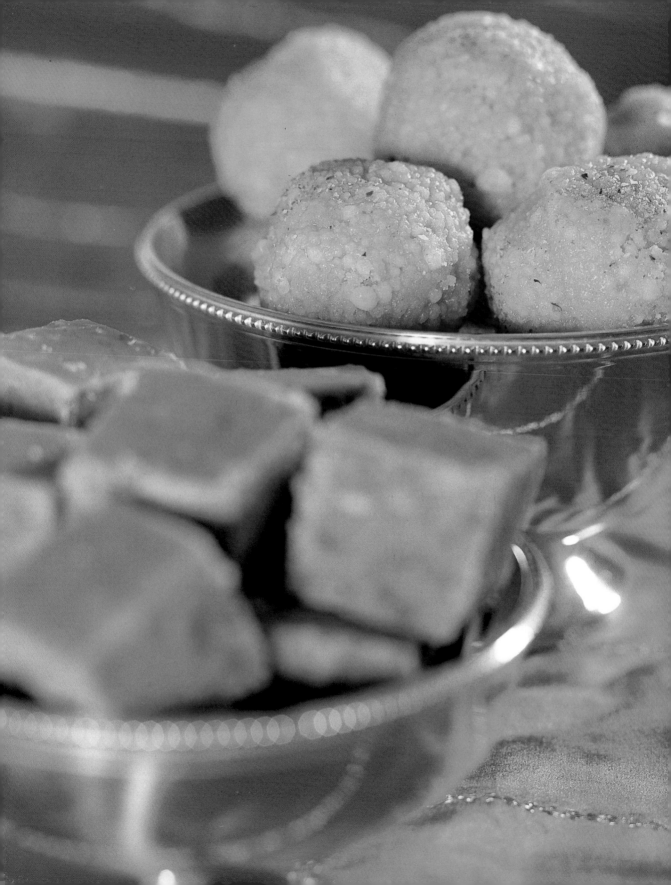

Towards the end of her pregnancy, the mother-to-be moves to her mother's house where, traditionally, the confinement takes place. Here another whirl of pampering begins. Often her marital home is in another city, so home-coming means that all her childhood friends will visit her to exchange gossip and news. They enjoy dressing their friend up, polishing her skin with sandalwood and cream, drawing henna patterns on her palms and feet and painting her nails with nail varnish. In the villages of north India the expectant mother is made to sit on a cushioned swing that is richly entwined with fresh flowers; she is embellished with bracelets, necklaces and a tiara of flowers while her friends sing and dance for her.

sweet balls or *ladoos* made of various ingredients including coconut, poppy seeds, fenugreek and edible gum. Some of these foods are also believed to improve the quality and quantity of breast milk. Fenugreek has the property of

'O woman! As this vast earth holds all these mountains, and does not let them fall when it revolves, so should your pregnancy be safe and a child be born in due course.' *prayer from the Artharva-Veda (between 900 and 500 BC)*

An expectant mother is encouraged to look after her health and her looks. Her most comfortable attire is the *salwar-khameez* a long, loose tunic worn over baggy, drawstring trousers. A scarf gracefully covers the burgeoning breasts and belly. I personally recommend this dress – it is elegant and comfortable and you will not grow out of it. The adjustable-waist trousers are a particular boon.

Traditionally, the new mother returns to her husband's home forty days after the birth. Soon after her baby is born, her mother cooks delicious, strengthening foods for her. In Punjab it will be *panjeeri*, a mixture of almonds, semolina and spices that provide energy. In the state of Maharashtra on the western coast, the new mother is given

toning the uterus after childbirth because it contains steroidal saponins, which resemble our sex hormones. The new mother is massaged with fragrant oils that will tone up her skin and bring her back to shape.

Pregnancy can be the perfect time to indulge yourself. People have few expectations of you, other than that you look after yourself. First pregnancy is also possibly the one time in adult life that you can call your own, away from the pressures of work and family. A new baby will change your life in ways that you never knew existed. If you live alone, it could be a time of introspection and planning. In the West, few women enjoy close family support as they do in India, so a woman must pamper herself. Keep a positive outlook, eat well, rest well and look and feel great. I end with a prayer from the Artharva-Veda, a collection of sacred hymns composed between 900 and 500 BC.

'O woman! As this vast earth holds all these mountains, and does not let them fall when it revolves, so should your pregnancy be safe and a child be born in due course.'

right
An assortment of delicious goodies such as these ladoos and squares of fudge are made to tempt and pamper an expectant mother.

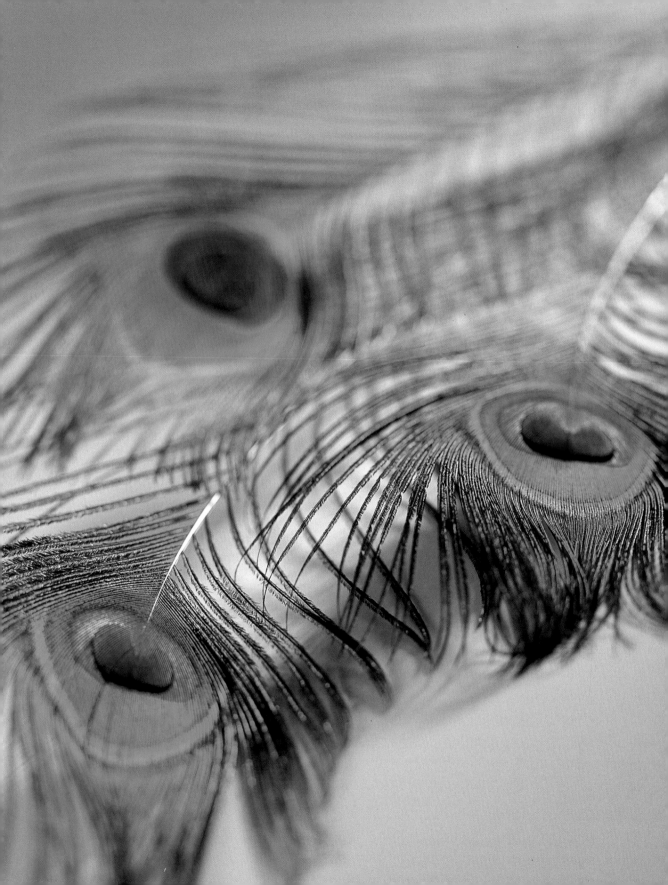

'When the season of rains, with its high clouds, has passed like youth, the earliest single kasa flower comes, like a grey hair on the earth.'

South Indian folk song

ageing

The concept of immortality and eternal youth is found in myths and legends the world over. The peacock, long considered the epitome of timeless beauty, is the subject of many such tales, and a peacock feather adorns the crown of the beautiful god Krishna as a symbol of his divinity. Where there is divinity, there is no age, no end. Indian alchemists, thousands of years ago, conjured up elixirs from gold, silver and mercury that were believed to prolong life, and even the gods went in search of that most exotic of eleixrs – *amrit*, or the nectar of immortality. The search is still continued today, with most medical research aimed at increasing the duration and quality of life.

All of us would like to look good for as long as possible. In our day-to-day life we do not even notice our first wrinkle or when the 'droop' begins. We take our bodies for granted and even get used to our body functions not per-forming to the best of their ability. As we grow older, we must listen to the voice inside more and more, become acquainted with our internal processes and walk to the beat of inner rhythms. In India our ancestors developed a social system whereby a person went through four stages of life depending on age. The third stage was *sanyasa* or renunciation. This meant that the person had to look beyond the material to the spiritual. Body rhythms were respected to fulfil religious aspirations. The internal systems were disciplined to focus the mind on the divine.

Traditionally, Indians have lived within the joint family. This is a system of communal living where the entire family, including distant relatives, all dwell under one roof. Each person has his or her own place in the infrastructure and there is a visible hierarchy. Indians have always revered the ancient or the old: photographs of dead ancestors are decorated with flower garlands, younger family members touch the feet and seek the blessings of older relatives before embarking on new ventures and their advice is sought on all matters including marriage or a choice of career. Most young Indians are happy to let their elders choose a life partner for them, taking into account family background, education, physical beauty and personal qualities. It is quite understood that younger members of the family will look after the older ones – emotionally as well as financially.

As growing Westernisation and work pressures influence the majority of people in contemporary India, the joint family is crumbling and more and more older people are beginning to live on their own. However, they are still well respected, honoured on festive occasions and cared for. They in turn fulfil traditional roles of responsibility, looking after grandchildren, passing on valuable knowledge and religious education and providing a support structure for their children who are most likely in the throes of their careers.

An older woman in India is given due respect and she becomes the genial, compassionate figure in her grandchildren's lives. According to custom, she has the liberty to dress up and adorn herself, sometimes as much as a newly-wedded woman, as long as her husband is alive. As a widow, however, she is expected to lead an austere life and turn her thoughts to spiritual pursuits. This gradual transition is taken for granted, as is the growing power that she may have due to her age and experience. She knows that ageing is inevitable and accepts that she will have to cope with changes. Society does not pressurise her to chase after the rainbows of youth and physical beauty alone. She is accepted for who she is.

My mother, now in her sixties, maintains that the elixir of vitality and beauty is found in sheer hard work. She says, 'Work as much as you can, for as long as you can and with as much devotion as you can. Your relationship with the work you enjoy will blow away tensions and unhappiness and make you beautiful, energetic and vivacious.' I think this is very sound advice. Work, as beauty expert Helena Rubinstein said in her nineties, keeps wrinkles out of the mind and the spirit.

below
While youth can admire the experience and wisdom of an older woman, age can also benefit from and enjoy the vitality and energy of youth.

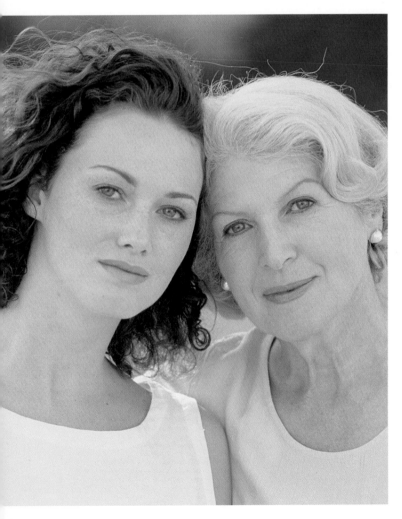

the body clock

Every age has its own plus points, compensations and promise of beauty. It also has its questions, trials and particular set of beauty queries.

teens Most people remember their teens with great affection. This is a time of gossiping with friends, of clandestine moments trying out mother's lipstick or perfume and of experimenting with new clothes and jewellery; it is full of the excitement of a new life opening up.

Your best asset here is sheer youth, summed up in an amusing Sanskrit saying that I heard a mother tell her daughter who spent most of her day in front of a mirror: 'Even a donkey looks good when it is sixteen years of age.' The sensible habits you develop in your teens will stand you in good stead in later life. Establish routines of cleansing and toning, of good dental care and body hygiene and, above all, work on your attitude to life. A happy approach to everything around you will reflect in your eyes and make you even more attractive.

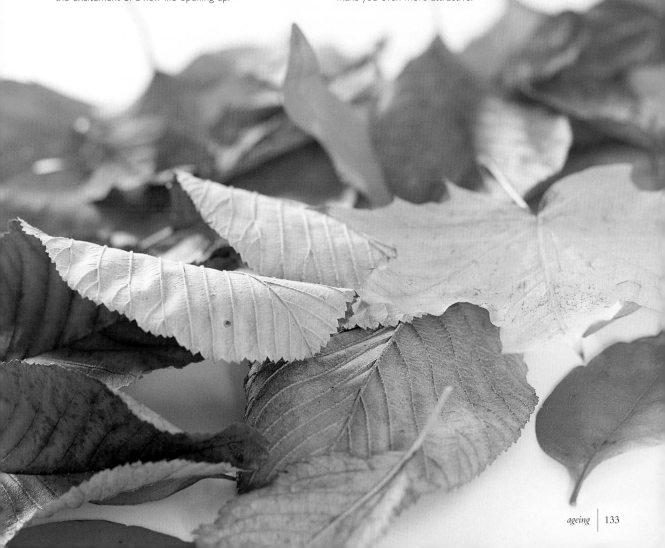

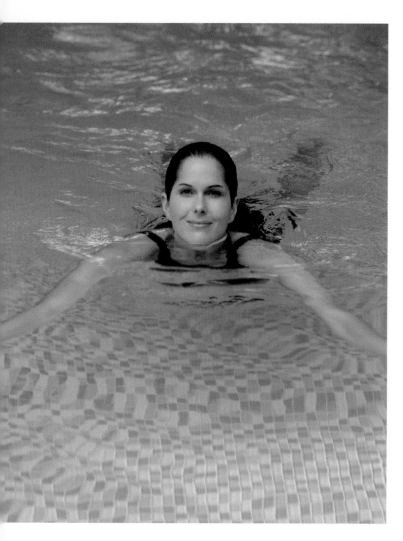

itself: cleanse and tone well and dab a little sandalwood paste on spots before going to bed. Protect your skin with sunblock every time you go out in the sun and make fitness and exercise a way of life.

the glowing years

The twenties, thirties and forties see a woman at her loveliest, when the individual nature of her skin and hair have become established. A woman at this stage is usually aware of what she wants from life and has the confidence and poise to present herself to the world.

A beauty routine is, however, still essential for maintenance. Stress, going on the Pill and constant travel can all take a toll on the skin and hair, so cleanse and moisturise regularly, using recipes that are suited to you. In our twenties many of us embark on a new career and looking our best at work is vital as well as professional. Pay attention to details – nails must be shaped and polished, the hair must be in good shape and the eyes and teeth should sparkle. Make-up for work should enhance your best features without being too heavy or obtrusive.

The thirties bring with them subtle changes announcing that the body is beginning to veer towards ageing. Fine lines appear, especially on dry skin, the muscles lose a bit of tone and the eyes begin to show signs of maturity. The pressures of raising a young family may

above
Seek out and pursue activities that both relax your mind and exercise your body. Swimming can be a particualrly therapeutic form of excercise.

Puberty is a disconcerting time of hormonal upheavals that can result in a spotty complexion, oily hair and excess weight. Wonderfully behaved baby skin can suddenly erupt into acne and you feel as if nothing you do will improve it. Remember not to camouflage pimples with make-up – they will only get worse. Deal with the problem not leave you much time for yourself, but prioritise yourself for a few minutes each day. You still want to look fresh and lovely and there is only one way to do that: work hard at it.

In her forties a woman's skin begins to lose some of its elasticity. The face and body start to sag and fine lines which appeared in the thirties grow deeper. This may be a time for a change of look – a hair tint or a new haircut, different make-up (as you grow older, make-up should also become more subtle) and perhaps a change of wardrobe. Fortnightly facials will go a long way in keeping the skin glowing and firm. If you have not done much exercise in the past, start now. Above all a smile and a twinkle in your eye will announce to the world that you are still young at heart and great fun to be with.

the fifties & beyond
Ageing really starts here. The skin receives less and less support from internal fat deposits and becomes loose and flabby. Lines develop into wrinkles and the colour of the skin becomes dingy. This can be corrected with massage and exercise, both of which boost the circulation and bring back the bloom to skin. Changes in production of oestrogen, the hormone responsible for menstruation and feminine curves, now cause all the wild and unexpected fluctuations associated with menopause. Even gentle exercise such as a walk in the fresh air or swimming will help you keep trim and energetic. The fresh exuberance of youth mellows but is replaced by the equally charming, rich patina of wisdom and experience. There is amazing grace in old age. No longer is there any pressure to be reed-thin; indeed a little filling-out looks flattering. The most important issue in old age is health and through good health comes natural beauty.

what to eat

Ayurveda also advises on what to eat and what to avoid from the age of fifty onwards. My grandmother always said that once the body begins to tell you that it is time, you should be prepared to alter your diet. A balanced meal with the six tastes of Ayurvedic nutrition helps to keep the elderly system in order. As you grow more mature, dieting is out of the question; instead eat regular, small meals throughout the day – with a good mix of starch, fats and proteins along with plenty of fresh fruit, vegetables. This aids the digestion, which may no longer be able to cope with large amounts. Ayurveda classifies food tastes in the following way:

1 *Sweet* – foods such as honey and sugar. This is considered a cooling taste, but should still be eaten carefully to

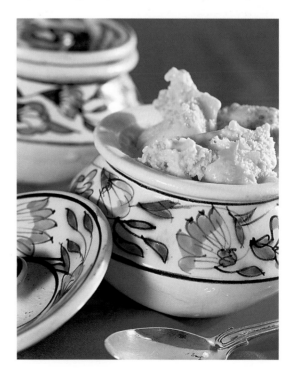

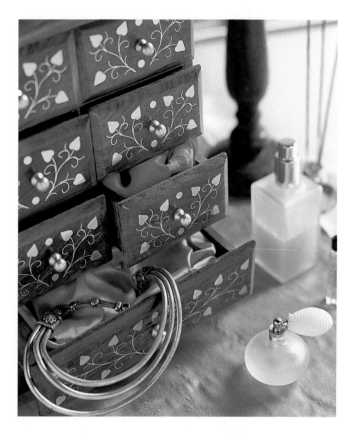

from premature baldness, grey hair and wrinkles of the skin.' Cut down on salt as you get older: remove the salt shaker from the table and choose fresh foods over processed ones.

4 *Pungent* – as in chillies, pepper and garlic. These can irritate a delicate digestion, so you should opt for blander foods whenever you can.

5 *Bitter* – few foods we eat are bitter. However, according to Ayurveda this taste is cleansing and aids digestion. Incorporate cumin seeds, coriander seeds or bitter herbs judiciously into your diet.

6 *Astringent* – this taste is cooling and comes close to being bitter, an example being turmeric. It is a healthy taste that is good for proper functioning of the internal organs.

pampering yourself

Old age almost always dries out the skin, making it leathery and more prone to wrinkles. Moisturise your skin well in the morning as well as at night. Do not forget your neck, hands and feet which show signs of age faster than the face. Tired skin will benefit from a weekly oatmeal scrub (see page 36). Freckles associated with age (liver spots) can be treated with a face wash of diluted lemon juice, or just rub with the cut side of half a tomato. If you have any over-ripe bananas, mash a few slices and apply all over the face and neck as an anti-wrinkle treatment. Wash off after twenty minutes.

above & far right
A traditional wood and inlay chest of drawers houses a private collection of secret potions, perfumes and jewellery that add to the feminine mystique. Every woman must have her own magic assortment.

avoid putting on excess weight. In Sanskrit the word *rasa* means both taste as well as emotion. These two are closely linked, so we often find ourselves eating sweets to compensate for the happiness we feel is missing in our lives.

2 *Sour* – foods such as lemon and yoghurt should be eaten in moderation as acids can lead to further acidity in old age.

3 *Salty* – this is a warming taste, although it causes the body to retain fluids. Charak writes in his treatise on Ayurveda, 'People who are accustomed to the excessive use of salt suffer

Treat the hair to a good oil massage. If you want a change of colour, do not use henna – it tends to turn white or blond hair bright orange. Tinting is an alternative, but there comes a point at which, when the hair turns silver or white, it is best to leave it natural. This looks extremely elegant and matches the change in complexion. Make-up should be pared down and clear; light colours such as corals, peach and pink should be chosen. Change the colour of your clothes, too, to complement your hair. Make the most of this time to read good books, listen to your favourite music and catch up with friends whom you have always wanted to see more often.

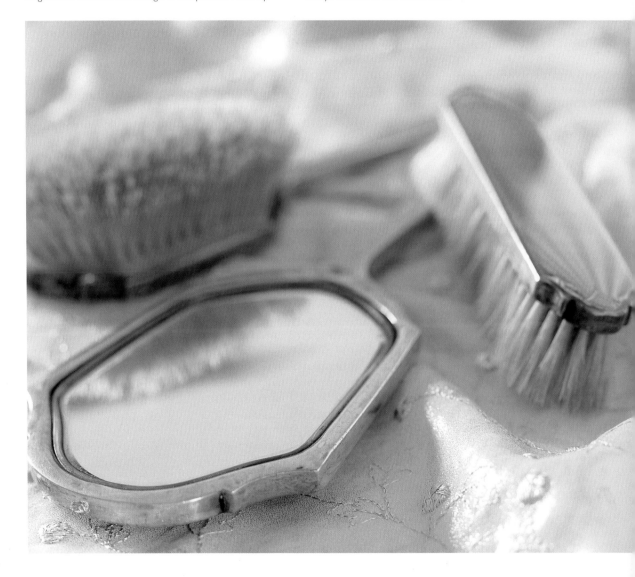

the menopause

When I was a child, weddings, festivals and Sundays would bring the entire coterie of my relatives together. In the afternoon, after a sumptuous feast, the women would shut themselves in a bedroom to rest for a while. Each child would snuggle up to a favourite aunt or grandmother and the chat sessions would start. Vital bits of information were exchanged, advice given and confessions made, and to me the entire process was delightfully secretive, warm and comforting. It made me feel special to belong to this womanly world that seemed so full of mysteries and incomprehensible magic.

'The change of life' was one subject discussed at these gatherings. From what was said, I gathered that at a certain point in life a woman had hot flushes or flashes where a burst of heat originating in the chest moved upwards, raising her body temperature uncomfortably. She might also experience dizzy spells, dryness in the vagina and feelings of tiredness and lethargy.

For most women, the change of life or menopause is the ultimate threshold between youth and age. Emotionally it is a time of upheaval when a woman may feel that because her ability to have babies is now gone, she is 'less of a woman'. Depression may follow, leaving her family to wonder what has suddenly happened to their loving wife and mother.

In India a lot of the heartache associated with the menopause is lessened by sharing the experience with other women. Older women recommend tried-and-tested techniques to others passing through this phase. A well-known remedy handed down in my family for vaginal dryness is to insert a swab of cotton wool

below

One of the most popular Indian fragrances is sandalwood, soul of this delightful sherbert.

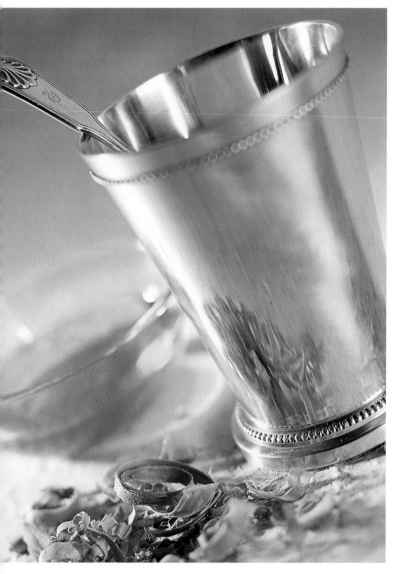

soaked in sesame oil every other night or at least for a few hours while you are resting. Be sure to wear a light sanitary towel to prevent staining. If sesame oil is difficult to obtain, you can use pure almond or olive oil.

Ayurveda has a miracle herb, *shatavari* or wild asparagus (*Asparagus racemosus*), for women going through the menopause. *Shatavari* in Sanskrit means 'one who possesses a hundred husbands': the rejuvenating action of the herb on the female reproductive organs is said to enhance youth and beauty and the capacity to have a hundred husbands. Two teaspoonfuls of the powdered root (available from Indian shops) is taken twice a day with half a cup of warm milk.

If, like countless women, you feel dizzy and tired, you must rest as much as possible to allow your body to adjust to changing circumstances. You are likely to experience bouts of tiredness, so it is important to slow down when you need to, perhaps even taking a short nap in the afternoon with the curtains drawn. Make yourself a glass of sandalwood sherbet, by mixing a pinch of fine sandalwood powder and a

It may also be worthwhile consulting your doctor about hormone replacement therapy (HRT), which some women claim makes them feel wonderful. There is a tendency during menopause to lose bone mass and many women suffer from a condition called osteoporosis where the bones become weak and brittle and can fracture easily. HRT helps to prevent osteoporosis and to maintain agility.

Positive thinking is the best antidote to the ills of menopause. Today's woman has technology, a career, a rich lifestyle and innumerable social extravaganzas and hobbies at her fingertips, and more than ever she is capable of taking her life in her own hands and shaping her destiny. One way of looking at the menopause, regardless of some of its drawbacks, is that it can be a time of great freedom – finally the monthly round of menstruation, which can hamper sport or travel, is over and there is no fear of unwanted pregnancies. Some women despair that a loss of periods will mean that they will be less feminine and there-fore less attractive. This is simply not true. A few wrinkles

'You herbs, born at the birth of time
More ancient than the gods themselves
You, who have a thousand powers...' *The Rigveda*

teaspoonful of honey in water. Alternatively try sandalwood syrup, which is available commercially. Sandalwood tones the reproductive organs, as does lemon balm, which may be easier to obtain. Make a tea with fresh lemon balm leaves, which have been used traditionally in Europe to relieve the pains of menopause. Lemon balm is reputed to calm the mind, rejuvenate the body and increase fertility.

and a wisp of grey hair will not, if you are worried, drive devoted husbands into the arms of a younger woman. Instead your inner beauty, experience and calm confidence will attract more people to you. But you will have to try hard to keep your spirits up and work on your beauty routine to give yourself the best possible start to a new and exciting chapter in your life.

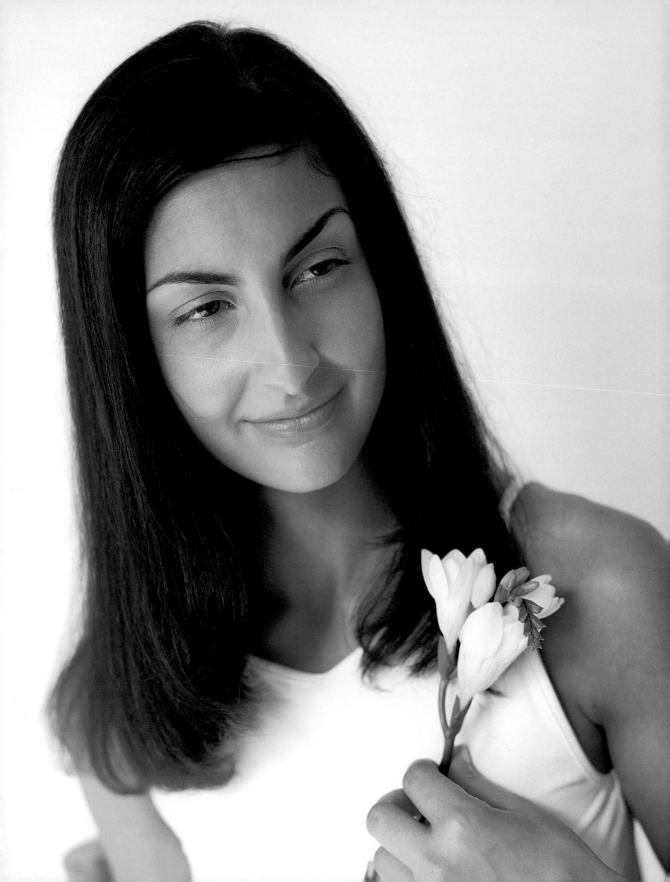

'I see your body in the sinuous creeper, your gaze in the startled eyes of deer, your cheek in the moon, your hair in the plumage of peacocks, and in the tiny ripples of the river I see your sidelong glances, but alas, my dearest, nowhere do I find your whole likeness.'

Meghadoot, written by Kalidasa between AD *375 and 455*

inner beauty

One of the strongest, most serene and perfectly collected women I have known in my life was my grandmother Uma. Hardly educated, married at the early age of twelve and thrust into full-blown family life when she was barely thirteen, she eventually grew into the pillar of the family, keeping everyone together and running the household with a firm but gentle hand. Even after she was widowed, which traditionally is a time when Hindu women retire to a life of religion, she carried on being her vivacious, generous self, bringing joy and comfort to everyone around her. She was the Robin Hood of the family, taking a bit from the wealthier members to pass on to those who were not so fortunate. Everyone loved her, me especially, and I often remember snuggling up to her at night, breathing her clean, 'old' smell and feeling perfectly safe and loved.

Inner beauty has nothing to do with physical appearance. A woman may not consider herself pretty, but if she has inner confidence, she is remembered long after she has left.

She leaves a mark wherever she goes and other women wish that they could be like her. In Sanskrit the word for a unique 'ownness' is *svabhava*. This implies that each person has an intrinsic disposition for which certain forms of living, livelihood, duties and behaviour are appropriate. Every person sets her own morals and has her own viewpoints and goes about life in tune with her inner needs and justifications. All religions teach us about a way of life where goodness prevails and we aim to commit ourselves to a perpetual endeavour of bettering ourselves.

I am convinced that a woman's life is more fraught with 'hurdles' than that of a man. Deep-rooted conditioning of what it means to be a woman still influences all of us, in spite of the fact that every kind of choice is available to many of us today. In Indian cities, as in the West, a girl can choose her own career; she can decide whether she wants to be married and to whom, whether or not to have children and how to live her life on her own terms.

Nonetheless it is still the woman who, once she has made her choice, will juggle her time, make sacrifices and compromises and ensure that her family is healthy and happy. The heady taste of personal freedom is often enjoyed only after the welfare of her partner and children has been attended to. Indians believe that a woman's strength and devotion to her family keep the unit stable and that her life and character set an example to her children. She ensures that the values and cultural traditions, both within the family as well as in the larger community, are carried on.

Many of the stresses of modern life are a result of our own perceptions. I once heard a wise man say, 'In times of personal conflict when faced with a situation which you don't agree with, ask yourself, "So what?" If your answer convinces you, act on it, if not, throw your negative feelings away.' This advice has held me in good stead and has helped me be anchored at the worst of times.

What I have learnt from my grandmother are lessons of personal courage, of overcoming adversity without compromising my ideals and complete generosity towards others. I

'the immortal goddess now has filled wide space, its depths and heights. Her radiance drives out the dark…' *Hymn in praise of the goddess of night*

However emancipated a woman might be, she is still aware of the importance of gentleness and generosity. Any woman who is excessively aggressive or hard is unbecoming and the feminist movement has realised this unchanging fact. A friend once remarked candidly, 'The true power of a woman lies in her ability to accept change. Being rigid is easy; having the grace and flexibility to alter her thinking gives her incredible strength…'

Patriarchal literature and jokes through the ages have often painted women as aggressive, jealous or malicious. All of us will agree that this is unfair, although feelings of envy seem to come more easily to women than to men, much as we might hate to admit it. Envy gets us nowhere; it only puts a bitter expression on an otherwise attractive face and twists the insides into knarled knots. It defeats a sense of self and makes us feel less than the object of envy. Surely it is better to banish these negative thoughts and cultivate a generosity of spirit which is so much more rewarding.

have seen that it pays to pursue one's dreams, but never at the cost of others. As my mother would say, 'No one can build a castle on the grave of another.' Leave envy, jealousy, lies and aggression well alone. Inner beauty can only shine through when you are at peace with yourself. For this you have to make the most of yourself – highlight the assets and work on the flaws. Be true to yourself and be at peace with yourself. There is no greater beauty than this. A hymn in praise of the Goddess of Night, has a message of generosity for us all: 'The immortal goddess now has filled wide space, its depths and heights. Her radiance drives out the dark…'

positive thinking

How many times have we admired a woman who walks into a room and glows with the radiance of a thousand suns? This woman is not merely gorgeous to look at. She is multidimensional and seems to have an aura of self-confidence, wit and humour with a sprinkling of justice and common sense. She has worked to rid herself of fear, self-doubt and nervousness and is happy to open herself to the world.

Every religion in the world teaches us that the face and body are reflections of what is inside. If we think unpleasant thoughts, it will show, whereas positive energies coursing through the heart and mind will bring an unparalleled radiance to the face.

Hinduism is based on a concept of *karma* or destiny, where human beings follow an ongoing cycle of self-realisation and improvement until the immortal soul merges with the Universal Being. Good thoughts and actions alleviate past sins and ease the path to salvation. Buddhists too believe in this theory of a cyclical birth process. Along with this doctrine comes the ability to accept that improving oneself is the only way to achieve long-lasting happiness. It is impossible to change anyone unless they themselves want to change. The only person that you have control over is yourself. Change yourself for the better and watch how everyone around you changes too.

The Buddhist doctrine of passive tolerance and *ahimsa* or non-violence can be followed at an emotional level as well. 'Live and let live' is a philosophy that can be learned and practised, and orthodox Buddhists will not utter a single harsh word to anyone, even if they are extremely angry. We are sometimes kinder to our pet animals than to the people around us. Better human beings are supremely aware of the value of mercy, forgiveness and kindness.

Hinduism, in a broad sense, upholds the teachings of *dharma*, a guide to the correct way of behaving. This is governed by a concept of rightness and regularity – the rising and setting of the sun, the seasons and harvest and even

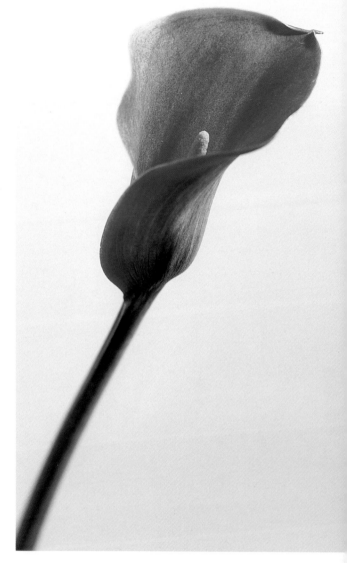

intrinsic justice which is a part of everything. The ancient texts known as the *Dharma-Shastras* lay down the precepts of social behaviour and an individual code of conduct based on justice, virtue, morality, religious merit and righteousness, law, duty, the good, the true, the way, the norm and the ideal. According to a hymn in the *Rigveda* 'Sweet are the winds to him who desires moral order.'

Islamic teachings are also based on concepts of self-development and goodness. One of the main tenets of

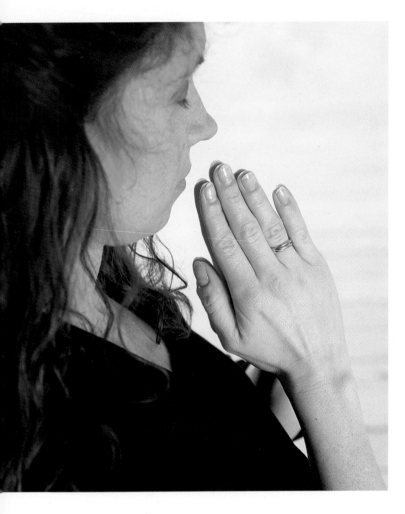

goodness. Have an implicit belief in your ability to make things better and they will be. I truly believe that if you pray for something good with all your energy, you have the magic within you to make it happen. Prayer concentrates your life force on something outside yourself and invites positive thoughts to yourself. If you are a non-believer, think about the beauty of nature – the flowers, fruits, landscapes and seasons which are so exquisite and magical. Focus on positive thoughts and absorb the qualities of your environment: the softness of a bird's wings, the tenderness of a young bud and the generosity of rain clouds. Believe in your self-worth and understand that the world is a happy place, made better because you are in it.

put others first

It is a material world we live in and it is all too easy to become self-centred and narcissistic. Although it is essential to be interesting (a sense of humour, an achievement that makes you proud of yourself and knowledge about what is going on in the world will help), it is important that you let others share their talents and glories with you as well.

Call up old friends and explore life together – you need not head for the once-in-a-lifetime trip to the Rajasthan desert; a trip to the local theatre or a concert will do. It will put a spark

above

The power of prayer must be experienced to be believed. Be thankful, wish for the best and enjoy the results of absolute communion with a higher force.

Islam is charity, where a spirit of selfless giving is encouraged. Muslims the world over donate personal wealth for the larger good of the community.

Whatever faith you follow, the most powerful force that you have inside you is prayer. Learn to pray every day, talk to your God and wish with all your might for truth, justice and into your existence and pull you out of a rut. If you feel dull and uninteresting, that is how you will appear to others. Instead, take up challenges, be daring and spontaneous and be strong enough to sometimes enjoy life like a child.

A good conversation consists of both superficial and serious dialogue. You must know how to listen as much as you should know what to say. It is of no use if you ask a question and then concentrate on someone across the room. The 'in-one-ear-out-the-other' habit is a very annoying one and will make you appear superficial and conceited. Some women blame the lack of time and having too many things on their mind. 'I'm too busy' has, I am told, replaced 'I love you' in many modern relationships. But then, every woman today is busy. Communicating with friends has become an instant process through e-mails, we speak of spending 'quality time' with children rather than quantity time, and we expect love relationships to crystallise overnight. If we feel that we are losing out because of the pace of life, a shuffling of priorities and better management of time is what we need.

Here are some suggestions to help you be a good listener:
1 Be really interested in what the other person has to say. It will give a perspective on how people think and will open new vistas for your own thought processes.
2 Never divide your attention while talking to someone. It is very unattractive, for instance, to have one beady eye on the television while trying to maintain a conversation. It is insulting, rude and totally unacceptable.
3 Assimilate what is being said so that you remember it next time. You will make someone's day if you recollect her favourite book or dream in life.

4 Absorb what you hear before deciding that you know better. An Indian saying that roughly translates as 'He picks up his tongue and touches it to the roof of the mouth,' describing those that speak without thinking, describes the kind of person you do not want to be.
5 Be compassionate. Sometimes a hug or holding a hand can convey far more than anything you say.
6 Learn the beauty of quiet togetherness. Silence is often more appropriate than incessant prattle and allows you to keep your ears open.

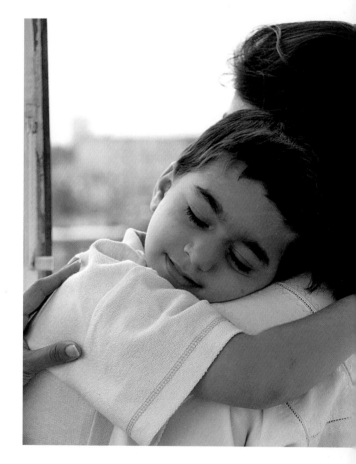

7 Cultivate your body language to show that you are interested. Face the person who is talking to you, maintain eye contact, 'open up' your stance and lean slightly forward.

8 Be generous with your expressions of sympathy, wonder, joy or pride and take a minute to form a good response.

busy schedule, stop and buy a tiny present for a friend. Share information, ideas and opportunities with loved ones and take the time to demonstrate your interest in and attraction to a husband or partner.

Give your time, energy, and love and you will receive in return, many times over. The reassurance and satisfaction inside will surely reflect on your face and in your personality.

make people feel special

Giving respect is equal to earning it. If you do not get along with certain people, it is best to leave them alone. Abusive language, petty quarrels or high-handedness get you nowhere and create a poor impression.

The cheapest and simplest way to make people feel special is to smile at them. Don't you love receiving a smile? Smiling takes a bit of courage – especially if you are timid and would rather retreat into your shell and not be noticed – but is well worth the effort. Someone who smiles easily looks more self-confidence and attracts people who are flattered to be sought out by your attention.

If you are social by nature, your task is simplified. Try to do small things for people you know. Always return telephone calls (it is just basic courtesy), phone to say 'thank you' or 'happy birthday' and offer condolences when appropriate. If you can find time in your

relaxation

Every woman needs to learn to relax – regardless of how busy her day is, and how indispensable she feels. For most women life passes in a whir of job, family and home and it constantly feels as though ten things, all equally important, are demanding her attention at once. These days many women opt for two to three careers at the same time, making relaxation a matter of survival.

I have often heard friends associate any relaxing activity with a sense of guilt: 'I should be taking the kids to music lessons instead of sitting in this sauna,' or 'I could have whipped up dessert for my husband in the time I've been watching this movie.' A woman is conditioned from childhood to think that she must nurture, nourish and navigate those around her to better times, sometimes at her own cost. In rural India a woman will spend her day collecting firewood, fetching water

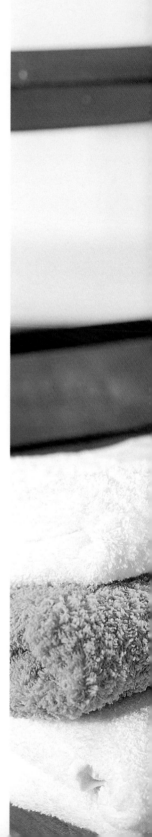

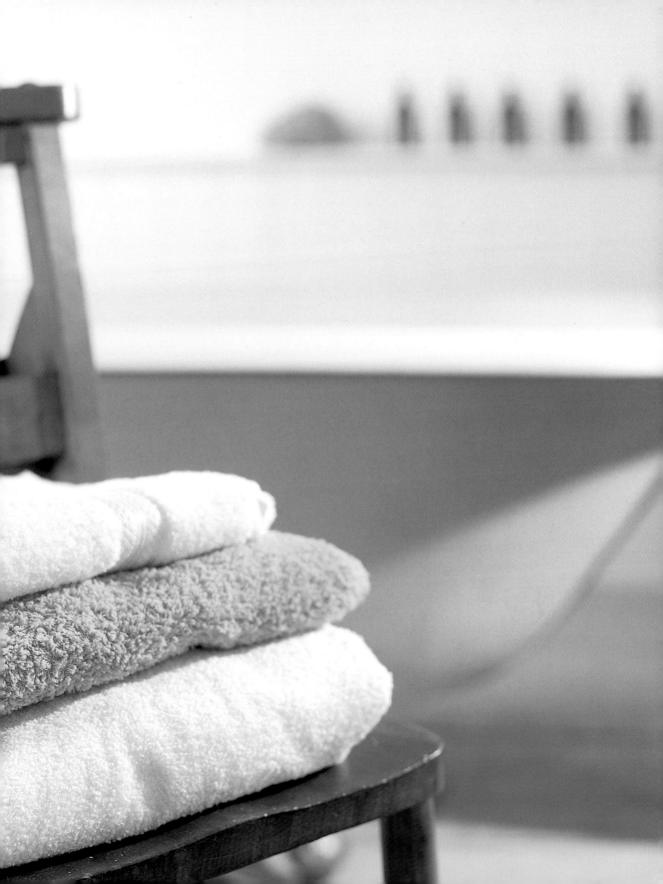

from a well, looking after children and cooking, and to top it all will feed her husband and children first and eat only if there is anything left. In spite of all this a woman is a woman first, a wife and mother second. If the stresses and pressures get to her, she will not make a good companion anyway. Relaxation is absolutely essential for beauty as stress only makes you wrinkled, grouchy and unhealthy.

You must relax even when the going is good. Use your lunch hour to take a walk in the fresh air or eat with a friend in the park. Lie down for ten minutes in the day, perhaps when you come home from work, and if you put on your favourite music you will be even more soothed. It may seem impossible to steal some time from the day for yourself, but consider it imperative and prioritise your work accordingly. Many women lose touch with their interests and hobbies once they get on to the treadmill of

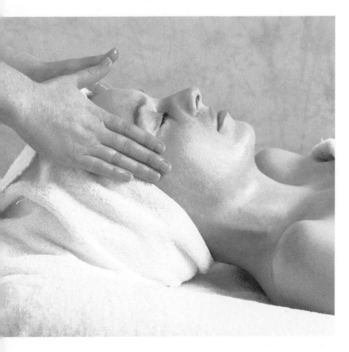

a career. Rediscover your love for books, art, theatre, movies, music, hand gliding, skating – whatever you love and will put the excitement of butterflies in your heart. If you are a young mother, use the afternoon when the baby is asleep to catch a nap for yourself.

When you are exhausted, a good massage is of tremendous help. According to an ancient Sanskrit verse, 'Just as a tree is nourished from its roots by watering, so also a person's strength increases with an oil massage.' You do not have to use oil every time. It helps to understand the *marmas* or ayurvedic pressure points, first mentioned in an ancient Hindu text, the *Atharva-Veda* (composed between 900 and 500 BC). Although these *marmas* coincide with the acupuncture points of traditional Chinese medicine, they cover a larger area rather than a point. One of the fathers of Ayurvedic medicine, Sushruta (AD 350), listed 107 *marmas* each with its own Sanskrit name. At the time, these points provided warriors and surgeons with vital information on where to strike the enemy or how to cure patients respectively. The knowledge of *marmas* is still used to stimulate or sedate the internal organs and promote health.

For quick relaxation try gently massaging these marmas:
1 *Gulpha* – the area where the bone juts out on the foot between the heel and the ankle.
2 *Jaanu* – the area on the knees roughly under the knee cap, extending to the back of the knees.
3 *Manibandh* – the entire region of the wrist.
4 *Kshipra* – the point on the palm under the index finger.
5 *Koorcha* – the point under the thumb.
6 *Indravastih* – the point between the wrist and the elbow.
7 *Asaha* – the points at the top of each shoulder.

8 *Krakarika* – the two points on either side of the spine at the back of the neck.

9 *Sthapni* – the point on the forehead between the eyebrows.

10 *Adhipati* – the spot at the centre of the top of the head.

Relaxation is a skill which must be developed if we are to cope sanely with the pace of modern life. However tempted we are to flop down in front of the television every night, it is far better to join a course, ring a friend or read to a child. Creative relaxation enriches the mind and calms the body.

sleep

We all take sleep for granted, sometimes under-estimating its contribution towards health and beauty. Most people need between six and eight hours of sleep a night. For truly relaxing and refreshing sleep, a good mattress is essential. A mattress that is too soft or too hard will give you backache and could lead to spine problems. An orthopaedic mattress or one that is filled with coconut fibre supports the back and ensures restful sleep.

Vastu shastra, the ancient Indian science of construction and decoration, is closely linked with nature. According to this it is unlucky to use a broken bed for obvious reasons; it may collapse. Further, it should be positioned so that your head points to the south and your

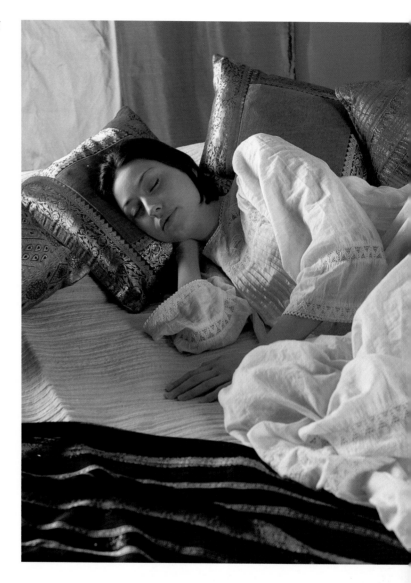

feet to the north. The reasoning behind this is that the body acts like a magnet with the head as the heaviest and most important part. If the head is towards the north, it will repel against the north pole of the earth, thus adversely

above & left

There is nothing quite as relaxing as sleep, even a quick nap can do wonders. A regular massage also helps to banish tension.

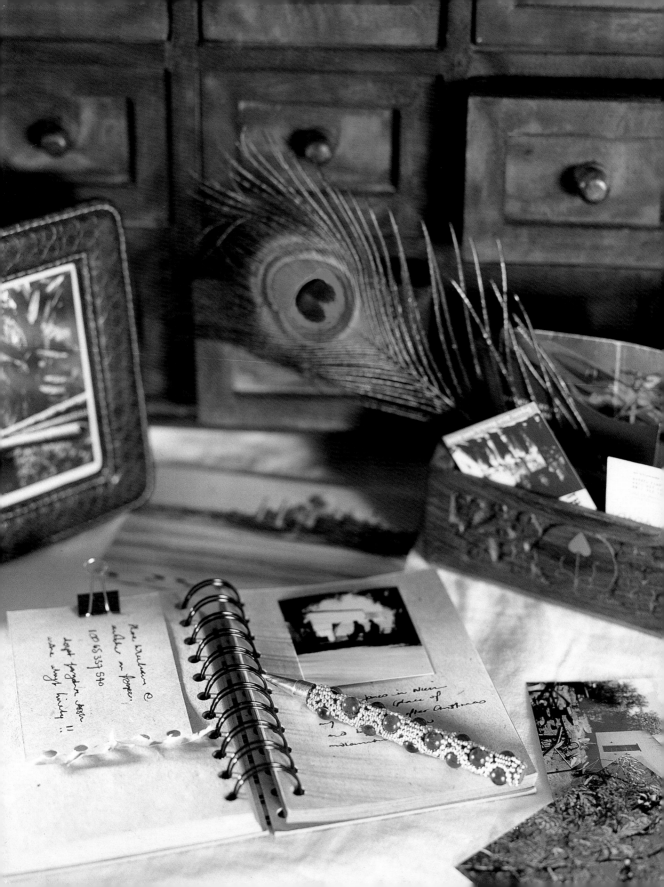

affecting blood circulation and therefore sleep.

The ancients believed that sleeping on the left side allows easy breathing from the right nostril, which is good for digestion and makes one healthy and outgoing, and open to sensuality and social exchange. Sleeping on the right side opens the left nostril more and this calms the system and brings it under control. Ayurveda forbids sleeping on the stomach as proper breathing is hampered.

ten tips for insomniacs

1 My grandmother's delightful remedy for sleeplessness was to make up a glass of warm milk with a pinch of ground turmeric (its antiseptic properties calm minor throat irritations and reduce phlegm which may keep you awake) and a little sugar. As a special treat she would drop in a dried fig that would nicely plump up with sweet milk to eat at the end. Milk has a high content of the amino acid tryptophan that seems to activate sleep-inducing chemicals in the brain, and its calcium content acts as a natural tranquilliser.

2 If you just cannot fall asleep, perhaps your body does not yet need the rest. Catch up on something else – write a letter, read a book or watch a boring programme on television, which in itself can be quite soporific.

3 A perfectly sensible piece of advice given to young mothers about fretful children works for adults too. Wake up an hour earlier each morning. Like the proverbial 'hyper' child, you will also nod off at bedtime.

4 If possible, elevate your feet slightly when you sleep – rest them on a fat pillow about 15cm (6in) above head level. The blood flows back from the feet towards the heart and this eases away excessive tiredness, which is an enemy of sleep.

5 Give the body time to wind down. Stimulation and sleep do not go well together. Cut back on stimulants such as alcohol, coffee, tea and colas which contain caffeine and 'pep up' the metabolism.

6 Try a warm bath with a few drops of relaxing essential oil such as rose, ylang ylang or orange blossom.

7 Be sure that the room is neither too hot nor too cold, that there is no light shining on to your bed and no disturbing noise keeping you awake. In rural India, where summers can be scorching, people make the most of the nights and sleep outdoors under a star-spangled sky.

8 My mother has an excellent solution, believing that a good day's hard work, after which the body is tired and the conscience clean, will soon put you to sleep naturally.

9 I have personally found that doing a spot of vigorous cleaning when I am especially restless calms me down. I am so tired aferwards that I am ready to drop and, best of all, I have a shiny, clean kitchen floor the next morning.

10 Another routine I follow is to pray just before I go to sleep. After my nightly beauty routine, I sit in bed for a while and converse with God, asking for guidance and strength and offering thanks for all that I have been given.

being a superwoman

Women all over the world are experiencing the heady taste of financial independence. In India this is more recent, but we are all coming to terms with the fact that more and more options are opening out before us. We travel, choose new and daring careers, decide what kind of partner to have and whether we want to have children. We are not afraid to fly to distant and exciting horizons and there has never been a better time to express oneself and be rewarded for one's assets. In the fields of education, law, medicine, nuclear science, beauty, marketing and finance women are at the fore, forging inspiring and sensational paths for the world to follow.

In India this liberation co-exists with tradition. Women will quite happily accept the training that begins in childhood, that they are nurturers and keepers of home fires. Indian women will explore the possibilities of their world, but never at the cost of their families. Although younger women are choosing to stay single as long as possible, there comes a time when everyone needs the finer emotions of love, trust and companionship to feel fulfilled. Getting married or having children are matters of personal choice, but I have yet to come across a woman who, for whatever reason, is unable to have a child and is happy about it. Ancient Indian texts such as the Vedas put this down to *prakriti* the intrinsic nature of women and their biological need to reproduce.

Family ties in India are very strong. The family shares work and takes joint responsibility for the upbringing of children. This unit runs smoothly mainly because of the women who, in their own way, collectively sort out emotional and financial problems (household finances are in their hands). There is a special sisterhood among the women of a family where the mother, her daughter and daughter-in-law and their children work together to ensure peace and harmony in the house. A great mother-to-daughter tradition flourishes in India. From childhood a girl is gently taught all it takes to make her an efficient housewife. She will watch her mother cook, make up traditional herbal medicines, deal with the vegetable vendor or laundry man, assist her father, keep accounts, socialise, beautify and dress herself and perform her *puja* or worship. No girl in India needs to be taught how to wear a *sari*; she just watches how her mother does it. Mothers and daughters can be best friends here – they are each other's confidante and moral support. A mother passes on beauty secrets and recipes to her daughter that have been jealously guarded by the family for many generations and she teaches her how to be a woman of the world.

In every country of the world, whether its women have technology at their fingertips or whether they go collecting berries in the bush, a woman's work is never done. Every woman knows that management of time is a skill worth learning if she wants to avoid being in a perpetual 'flap'. Serene and beautiful seems the woman whose life runs like clockwork. She is elegantly groomed, flourishing in her career, her love life and children are perfect and she is a witty and confident party-goer. But behind this glamour, this woman undoubtedly has mastered the art of time and energy management. She is clued up about how much time to allot to a task, when and how much to delegate, how to relax and how to please everyone around her. She knows that she cannot afford the addictions of modern life – drug abuse, excess alcohol, smoking – as these are all detractors from health and beauty. She is aware that she does not need these crutches to appear liberated or smart; she has the power of her own mind and her personality to achieve that. For her an active, disciplined and successful life is a perpetual high; she is not looking for instant boosts that are shallow and transient.

A superwoman knows that life is too short and it is possible to do countless things at the same time if you are an efficient manager. Today's woman works, in some instances at two or three careers, manages her house and children, keeps in touch with friends and looks happy and full of life. Her love for life is addictive and she touches everything around her with a special magic. This superwoman is not someone we only read about or see on television. She lurks inside each of us, waiting to emerge, wanting to drink in life in great gulps and experience the thrill of beauty and generosity. Let your special lady out: she will set you gloriously free.

managing time & family

One of the most amazing women I know is Rajam. For thirty years she worked in the heart of Bombay, rising each day at 5a.m. to store up water (in many places in India, municipal water is supplied for only an hour or two each day), fix breakfast and pack lunch for her husband, two children and herself. Then she would drop the kids off at school and stand for an hour on a smelly, crowded train as it chugged in from the suburbs to the city centre. At the

end of the day this journey would be repeated. Once home, dinner had to be cooked and the family fed; plates had to be rinsed and clothes washed. In spite of all this, I never once saw Rajam without her trademark grin which wrinkled her eyes and showed her even, white teeth. She was extremely generous with her time (in spite of a maddening lack of it), affectionate without fault and never expected anything in return. Rajam strikes me as a 'complete sou', someone who is like the lotus mentioned in the Hindu religious text, the Bhagvad-Gita, which is ethereal and perfect, although it lives only in slimy and wretched water.

From time to time, things will crop up in life to shake your sense of equilibrium. Sometimes these disturbances are fleeting, at other times they can turn your life upside down. If you see beyond the obvious to what you really want and are willing to work hard to achieve it, you can overcome almost any obstacle. Remember that you alone are responsible for your actions and are, at the end of the day, in charge of your destiny.

Here are some hints to help you to manage your time:

1 However ambitious or energetic you are, accept what is possible during a given time period and what is not, to avoid the disappointment of failure later.

2 Avoid unnecessary stresses. Letting go of unimportant issues takes courage and strength of heart. Petty jealousies, fights, arguments and addictions such as smoking or drug-taking all lead to negativity that will eat into your precious time.

3 Prioritise your work: this may sound like a cliché, but how many times do we flutter about doing things that could easily be done later, sometimes pushing urgent tasks to the back burner?

4 While certain things in life change and provide variety, it is essential to work these around set routines which stabilise and anchor your life. Constant change is distracting and you get the feeling that you are never able to finish anything that you start.

5 To be an efficient time manager, you have to be a good 'people' manager first. Treat people well and they will love you for it. They will be willing to give you their time, take over some of your tasks and help you towards your goals. At the very least there will be smiling faces all around you, which in itself is inspiring.

6 Write down lists of appointments and work that needs to be done in the day. Tick off each item as you complete it. At the end of the day a row of tick marks is incredibly satisfying and you know that you have worked through the list in an efficient, organised manner. Similarly, use post-its, a diary, a dictaphone… whatever it takes, as reminders to yourself.

7 However busy you are, set aside time for yourself and see this as essential and not as an indulgence.

8 Every child needs its mother's approval. It helps them to become more confident and independent if you are relaxed and accept that they can look after themselves. Some women take the dictatorial rule of 'mother knows best' so far

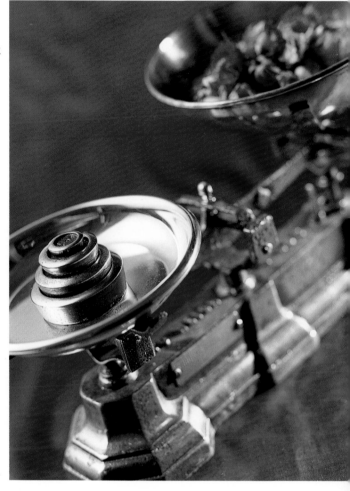

You are the remover of inaction and laziness O sacred Saraswati You are worshipped by Brahma, Vishnu and Mahesh, Please protect and energise me. *Sanskrit prayer to Saraswati, the goddess of knowledge*

that they end up stifling both their children and themselves.

9 Make sure that you communicate with your children. They understand a great deal more than we give them credit for and are usually reasonable enough to understand the demands of your life. In fact, you can make them into your allies, allowing them to assist you in small chores.

10 Try to spend quality time with your partner each day. It is important to nourish and enrich your relationship if it is to sustain and flower. Keep the romance going and do not allow yourself to become jaded. If you once wrote him love-notes or telephoned him at his office in the middle of day, try reviving these. Romantic routines are boring; love surprises are magic.

11 Try to gather as much goodwill as possible from your extended family by being good to them. They will love you, help you, look after your children and provide you with an incredible support system. Keeping up with the entire family may be too time-consuming, so start with one or two relatives and watch how the network attracts more members into it.

being a single parent

Indian mythology is full of heroines who have raised their children single-handedly to be brave and valiant. Foremost among such stories is that of Shakuntala who, after being rejected by her husband the king because of a sage's curse, went back to the forest where she had been brought up. There she gave birth to a son and raised him to be strong and fearless. A few years later the king, who by then realised his folly in allowing Shakuntala to leave, was riding past the forest when he saw a young boy playing with a couple of frisky lion cubs. Astonished at such courage in one so young, the king went up to the boy to ask him who he was. This child was Bharat, the son of Shakuntala and King Dushyant, who was to be one of India's greatest

monarchs and after whom India was named. (One of the many names of India in many local languages is Bharat.) Needless to say, Dushyant took Shakuntala and Bharat back to his kingdom with great pomp and celebration.

The modern woman seems to be at a crossroad. It is no longer a stigma to be divorced or a single parent (in India it was till quite recently – the late 1980s). However, looking after children on your own and raising them to be good human beings while earning a living and running a home is not easy. The demands on your time and energy are endless. Managing your time around your children is the topic for another book, but here are a few bits of advice I have collected from the wise, old Indian grannies I know:

1 Pull down your own level of hypertension. Children will be children, they will scream, make a mess, eat things that have fallen on to the floor or destroy your paper work. It would be impractical to say that you should turn a blind eye to everything, but little things should be put down to babyhood. Unless it is destructive to their health, consider that they are clearing their lungs, learning to handle objects, acquiring immunity from infection or enjoying the sound of tearing paper!

2 Mealtimes can be extremely stressful. A baby will usually eat only what it wants. If your doctor says that the child is healthy, do not spend hours on force-feeding, shouting, threatening or chasing your child.

3 Disciplining a child grows more and more difficult in an age when television and other media are constantly throwing conflicting images at them about how to behave. Accept that your children can never be you – they are the people of their own new world – but set down a list of rules that they absolutely have to abide by. Too much control or too much 'give' both have the same end result: badly brought-up children.

4 Build up your support systems. Enlist the help of your relatives and friends to look after your children sometimes and give them a sense of family. This network has been successful in Indian family life and is slowly being lost as people move far away from each other for work reasons.

5 Let your children play in the open air. Excess energy will be burnt off, the wind and sun will dance on their skin and hair and they will be relaxed and tired at the end. They will also be out of your way, while you catch up on jobs that need doing.

6 Keep a close watch on the company your children keep. Older children need their peers' approval and to be seen as fitting in with their crowd. It will help if you are more a friend than a nagging critic.

7 In the midst of all this, however impossible it may sound, make time for yourself. Relax, meet a friend, do your nails or whatever, so that you retain a sense of self. Involve your children in your hobbies – teach them the intricacies of music, dance or opera, read them the news, let them observe your world and how you function because you are the most powerful example that they will follow.

8 Your children are individuals who will follow their own destiny as you must yours. When the time comes, let them fly free without

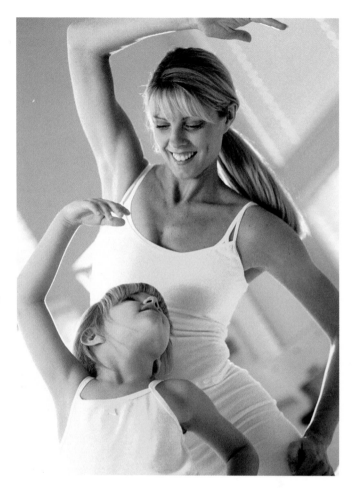

expecting them to provide an anchor to your own life.

In a scenario of stress, women tend to first look into themselves to see if they are at fault and will all too easily take the blame. Work towards absolving yourself of guilt. Everyone should be responsible for their own actions and all you can do is be true to yourself.

above

Children are soft, fragrant and innocent. Their company can be very energising and refreshing. Look at the world through their eyes and you will never feel old.

index

Entries in **bold** denote a recipe and numbers in **bold** denote a picture.

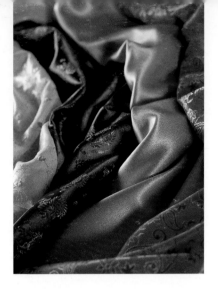

acknowledgements

As always a big *namaste* to Kyle Cathie for saying yes to this book, to Kate Oldfield, and to Sheila Boniface for her unbound enthusiasm and hard work. A tip of the hat to Teresa Chris, my agent and friend, for being constant and bright, to my mother Vimla Patil, for anecdotes and recipes, to the family of female relatives for their excited advice through the years and to friends and acquaintances who shared their valuable secrets so freely. A big kiss to my late grandmother Uma who is surely smiling down at me from her heavenly home and a big hug to my husband Nitish and my two flowers Arrush (*aged 4*) and Saayli (*aged 2*) for excusing me from so many (*and in India, they are endless!*) family engagements while I wrote, wrote, wrote!!!

bibliography

Herbs for Health and Beauty, Suman Seth, India Book House Publishers, 1996

Medicinal Plants, Dr. S.K. Jain, National Book Trust, 1968

The Piper Book of Beauty, Chodev, Piper Books, 1979

Herbal Remedies and Home Comforts, Jill Nice, Orient Paperbacks, 1990

Celebrations, Vimla Patil, IBH, 1994

Hindu World, Vol. 1 and 2, Benjamin Walker, Indus, 1995

Hindu Samaskaras, Rajabali Pandey, Motilal Banarisidas Publishers, 1994

Vogue Complete Beauty, Deborah Hutton, Octopus Books Ltd, 1983

credits

Aargee Novelties Concord Business Centre Concord Road Acton London W3 0TJ (020 8896 0500)

Dhaminis 277A Green Street London, E7 (020 8503 4200)

India Jane 140 Sloane Street London SW1X 9AY (020 7730 1070)

Neal Street East 5 Neal Street Covent Garden London WC2H 9PU (020 7240 0135/6)

The Hive Honey Shop 93 Northcote Road London SW11 6PL (020 7924 6233)

Models and make-up artists

Naren, Monica, Zoë, Illary, Chrissy (Angels Model Agency), Alex, Kate and Stephanie

Photography

Superstock: p114 (Florian Fanke) and p157 (Jiang Jin)

Telegraph Colour Library: p9 (Peter Adams), 10 & 24 (J.P.Fruchet), 27 (Tipp Howell) and 132 (Paul Viant)

Laura Hodgson p19, 72 & 134 and The Dorchester Spa p148